TOGETHER WE ARE STRONGER

AF696437

2007 Membership Application full year

01700E

Yes.

I accept your invitation for a full-year membership in the American Medical Association.

Members who reside in Oklahoma and Mississippi must join directly through their state or county medical society.

A physician or medical student who applies for direct membership in the AMA is encouraged to also join his/her state and local medical societies.

Legal first name | Middle name | Legal last name

Maiden name | Suffix

Street (Where you want your membership materials delivered. **Cannot** mail to school mailrooms or P.O. Boxes)

City | State | ZIP

ME# or birth date (*to aid in tracking/identification*)

Send me weekly e-mails about AMA advocacy initiatives, members-only surveys and other breaking news. My e-mail is:

Daytime phone | E-mail address

Students only:

Medical school (*International students are not eligible for membership until graduation.*) | Expected grad year

Method of payment (*see rate chart below*)

____Check (*Please make your check payable to: American Medical Association*)

____Please charge my: ☐ Visa ☐ MasterCard ☐ American Express

Please check credit card payment method below: (**See back for credit card payment information.*)

❑ 1. Credit card single payment

Options 2 & 3 below are recommended.*

Available to regular, military and fully retired membership categories only.

❑ **2. Credit card single payment with automatic renewal**

❑ **3. Credit card installment payment with automatic renewal**

Account number | Expiration date ____________

Cardholder's signature ____________________

Full-year membership

____$420 Professional practice

____$315 Second year in medical practice

____$210 First year in medical practice

____$280 Military

____$210 Semi-retired

(65 and over, working 1-20 hours a week)

____$ 84 Fully retired

Intern/resident/fellow

____$ 45 One-year membership

____$120 Three-year membership

____$160 Four-year membership

Medical student

____$20 One-year membership

____$38 Two-year membership

____$54 Three-year membership

____$68 Four-year membership

Three easy ways to join:

Return the application to:

Membership Processing
American Medical Association
P.O. Box 4188
Carol Stream, IL 60197-9791

(800) 262-3211

www.ama-assn.org/go/join

(*continued on page 2*)

Applying for AMA membership

Conditions of AMA membership and application
Membership is contingent upon the American Medical Association's (AMA) acceptance of the membership application. The endorsement, deposit or negotiation of an applicant's check does not guarantee admission into or acceptance of membership by the AMA. Checks received will routinely be deposited without a determination of the propriety of the payment or the applicability of the amount. Applicants who are not admitted to membership will receive a refund from the AMA for the amount submitted.

Compliance with the Principles of Medical Ethics as interpreted in the Code of Medical Ethics, the Bylaws of the American Medical Association, and the Rules of the AMA Council on Ethical and Judicial Affairs are conditions of applying for AMA membership.

- The Principles are a declaration of ethical guidelines, created by the AMA for physicians and are accessible online at *www.ama-assn.org/ama/pub/category/2512.html*.
- The Code of Medical Ethics may be viewed online at *www.ama-assn.org/ama/pub/category/2498.html*.
- The AMA's Bylaws are accessible at *www.ama-assn.org/ama/pub/category/13374.html*.
- The Rules of the Council on Ethical and Judicial Affairs are available at *www.ama-assn.org/ama/pub/category/13375.html*.

Unless otherwise disclosed to the AMA Office of General Counsel, **by submitting your application you confirm you have not:**

(i) been convicted of a fraud or a felony within the last five years;
(ii) had any action taken against you in any jurisdiction within the last five years (or extending to within the last five years) regarding your license to practice medicine (including actions involving revocation, suspension, limitation, probation or any other sanctions or conditions imposed upon your license); or
(iii) been the subject of any disciplinary action by any medical society, hospital staff, federal or state government within the last five years.

The Health Care Quality Improvement Act requires professional societies (such as the AMA) to report certain professional review actions, including denial of membership, to the National Practitioner Data Bank. Illinois law governs any legal matter relating to membership decisions by the AMA.

Credit card payment information

***Credit card options:** (1) Single payment available to all members. (2) Single payment with automatic renewal, and (3) Installment payment with automatic renewal applies to regular, military and fully retired membership categories only.

Pay monthly. Installment payments begin the month payment is received and are paid in full by Dec. 31, 2007. Renewal of both automatic payment options will be charged in January 2008, with one lump sum for single payment and 1/12 of the annual fee for installment payments.

Participation in either of the two automatic renewal options ensures continuity of your membership benefits and helps save your AMA valuable resources. With the automatic renewal options, your membership will continue from year to year unless cancelled by either party. The AMA guarantees it will not change your future membership dues without prior written notice.

FA12:06-0417:6/06

American Medical Association Contact Information

American Medical Association
515 N State St, Chicago, IL 60610 312 464-5000
www.ama-assn.org

Membership information
800 262-3211 msc@ama-assn.org
www.ama-assn.org/go/membership

Adolescent health
312 464-5315 gaps@ama-assn.org
www.ama-assn.org/go/adolescenthealth

Allied health education
312 464-5333 dorothy.grant-bryant@ama-assn.org
www.ama-assn.org/go/alliedhealth

AMA Foundation
312 464-4200 kathleen.macarthur@ama-assn.org
www.amafoundation.org

Becoming an MD
becominganmd@ama-assn.org
www.ama-assn.org/go/becominganmd

Continuing medical education
312 464-4671 cme@ama-assn.org
www.ama-assn.org/go/cme

Council on Ethical and Judicial Affairs
312 464-4823 ceja@ama-assn.org
www.ama-assn.org/go/ceja

Council on Medical Education
312 464-4515 barbara.barzansky@ama-assn.org
www.ama-assn.org/go/councilmeded

Council on Scientific Affairs and Public Health
312 464-5046 nancy.nolan@ama-assn.org
www.ama-assn.org/go/csa

Domestic violence
312 464-5476 violence@ama-assn.org
www.ama-assn.org/go/violence

Fifth Pathway
312 464-4662 marina.ramos@ama-assn.org
www.ama-assn.org/ama/pub/category/9306.html

Find a residency or fellowship
312 464-4748 rfs@ama-assn.org
www.ama-assn.org/ama/pub/category/6920.html

FREIDA Online
800 266-3966 freida@ama-assn.org
www.ama-assn.org/go/freida

Genetics and molecular medicine
312 464-4964 lawrence.o'connor@ama-assn.org
www.ama-assn.org/go/genetics

Gifts to physicians from industry
312 464-4668 rabia.akram@ama-assn.org
www.ama-assn.org/go/ethicalgifts

GME data requests
312 464-4487 sarah.brotherton@ama-assn.org

GME Directory
312 464-5333 enza.perrone@ama-assn.org
www.ama-assn.org/go/mededproducts

GME E-letter
312 464-4635 gme@ama-assn.org
www.ama-assn.org/go/gmenews

Health literacy
312 464-5357 barbara.correll@ama-assn.org
www.amafoundation.org

Infectious Diseases
312 464-4147 www.ama-assn.org/go/infectiousdiseases

Liaison Committee on Medical Education
312 464-4933 www.lcme.org

Medical education books and CDs
312 464-5333 enza.perrone@ama-assn.org
www.ama-assn.org/go/mededproducts

Medical Education Bulletin
312 464-4693 sylvia.etzel@ama-assn.org

Medical licensure
312 464-4635 fred.lenhoff@ama-assn.org
www.ama-assn.org/go/licensure

National GME Census
800 866-6793 gmetrack@aamc.org
www.aamc.org/gmetrack

Program director mailing labels
312 464-4693 sylvia.etzel@ama-assn.org

State-level GME data
312 464-4659 jacqueline.edwards@ama-assn.org

Virtual Mentor
312 464-5438 virtualmentor@ama-assn.org
www.virtualmentor.org

AMA Sections/Interest Groups; AMA Advocacy Agenda

The AMA represents you: Join today

The AMA offers many sections and special groups representing all physicians. All members receive the *Journal of the American Medical Association* and *American Medical News*. To join the AMA, call 800 AMA-3211, access www.ama-assn.org/go/join, or complete the attached membership form.

Gay, Lesbian, Bisexual and Transgender (GLBT) Issues Advisory Committee
312 464-5722 glbt@ama-assn.org
www.ama-assn.org/go/glbt

Group Practice Physicians Advisory Committee
312 464-4546 carrie.waller@ama-assn.org
www.ama-assn.org/go/imgs

International Medical Graduate Section
312 464-5622 img@ama-assn.org
www.ama-assn.org/go/imgs

Medical Student Section
312 464-4746 mss@ama-assn.org
www.ama-assn.org/go/mss

Minority Affairs Consortium
312 464-4392 mac@ama-assn.org
www.ama-assn.org/go/mac

Organized Medical Staff Section
312 464-2461 omss@ama-assn.org
www.ama-assn.org/go/omss

Resident and Fellow Section
312 464-4978 rfs@ama-assn.org
www.ama-assn.org/go/rfs

Section on Medical Schools
312 464-4655 section@ama-assn.org
www.ama-assn.org/go/sms

Senior Physicians Group
312 464-5728 spg@ama-assn.org
www.ama-assn.org/go/spg

Women Physicians Congress
312 464-4392 wpc@ama-assn.org
www.ama-assn.org/go/wps

Young Physicians Section
312 464-4978 yps@ama-assn.org
www.ama-assn.org/go/yps

2006 AMA Health Care Advocacy Agenda
The AMA will help doctors help patients by focusing on:

Medical liability reform
To preserve patients' access to care, the AMA will continue to lead an aggressive, multi-year campaign to reduce medical liability premiums:

- At the federal level, the AMA is fighting in Congress for MICRA-like reforms, including a $250,000 cap on non-economic damages in medical liability cases.
- At the state level, the AMA is providing resources to support similar state reforms.

Medicare physician payment reform and regulatory relief
As the leading force in Washington for Medicare reform, the AMA will be relentless in the battle to replace the flawed Medicare physician payment formula. The AMA will also push Congress and federal agencies to reduce costly and counter-productive administrative burdens and to eliminate unfunded mandates, which interfere with access to quality care for America's seniors.

Expanding coverage for the uninsured and increasing access to care
The AMA is committed to leading the response of America's physicians to solve the health coverage crisis for all uninsured patients:

- In the short term, the AMA will strongly advocate for incremental measures to expand coverage for children and lower income families and individuals. Further, the AMA will work to build political pressure for action on both coverage and access to care.
- In the long term, the AMA will continue to press for the adoption of a consumer-driven, market-based plan to expand coverage through tax credits and insurance market reforms.

Improving the health of the public
The AMA will provide effective programs and tools to help doctors improve the health of the public around:

- *Healthy lifestyles*—provide tools for physicians and advocate for national policies that help improve patient behaviors around obesity, tobacco, and alcohol.
- *Health disparities*—help physicians reduce racial and ethnic disparities in health care and health status.
- *Disaster preparedness*—develop training programs to help physicians and their communities prepare for disasters and to equip them to provide an effective medical response.

Patient safety and quality improvement in health care
In 2005 the AMA led the passage of the Patient Safety law. In 2006 the AMA will continue to lead physicians' efforts to measurably improve patient safety and quality of care by:

- Working to ensure the law's implementation and to advance other measures, including voluntary reporting systems with strong confidentiality protections.
- Continuing to convene the highly respected Physician Consortium for Performance Improvement to develop evidence-based performance measures to improve the quality of care.

Managed care reform
The AMA will continue to combat third-party interference with the physician-patient relationship, including advancing anti-trust reform; eliminating unnecessary hassles and unfair payment practices; and fighting for reimbursement decisions that are based on optimal patient care, not economics.

Medical Licensure and Medical Education Organizations

Accreditation Council for Graduate Medical Education
515 N State St
Chicago, IL 60610
312 755-5000 312 755-7498 Fax
www.acgme.org

American Board of Medical Specialties
1007 Church St, Ste 404
Evanston, IL 60201-5913
847 491-9091 847 328-3596 Fax
www.abms.org

American Hospital Association
One N Franklin
Chicago, IL 60606
312 422-3000 312 422-4796 Fax
www.aha.org

Educational Commission for Foreign Medical Graduates
3624 Market Street
Philadelphia, PA 19104-2685
215 386-5900 215 386-9196 Fax
www.ecfmg.org

Federation of Medical Licensing Authorities of Canada
Sylvia Smith, Executive Secretary
2283 St Laurent Blvd, PO Box 8234
Ottawa, ON K1G 3H7
613 738-0372 613 738-9169 Fax
www.fmlac.com

Federation of State Medical Boards of the United States
PO Box 619850
Dallas, TX 75261-9850
817 868-4000 817 868-4099 Fax
www.fsmb.org

Joint Commission on Accreditation of Healthcare Organizations
One Renaissance Blvd
Oakbrook Terrace, IL 60181
630 792-5000 630 792-5005 Fax
www.jcaho.org

National Association Medical Staff Services
2025 M St, NW
Washington, DC 20036
202 367-1196 202 367-2196 Fax
www.namss.org

National Board of Medical Examiners
3750 Market St
Philadelphia, Pa 19104-3102
215 590-9500 215 590-9555 Fax
www.nbme.org

National Board of Osteopathic Medical Examiners
8765 W Higgins Rd, Ste 200
Chicago, IL 60631-4101
773 714-0622 773 714-0631 Fax
www.nbome.org

National Committee for Quality Assurance
2000 L St NW, Ste 500
Washington, DC 20036
202 955-3500 202 955-3599 Fax
www.ncqa.org

National Practitioner Data Bank and Healthcare Integrity and Protection Data Bank
PO Box 10832
Chantilly, VA 20153-0832
800 767-6732
www.npdb-hipdb.com

Royal College of Physicians and Surgeons of Canada
774 Echo Dr
Ottawa, Ontario, K1S 5N8
800 668-3740 613 730-8830 Fax
http://rcpsc.medical.org

United States Medical Licensing Examination (USMLE)
3750 Market St
Philadelphia, PA 19104-3190
215 590-9700 215 590-9470 Fax
www.usmle.org

Assessing medical education and career options?
Beginning a residency or practice?
Considering a career change?
Determining whether to relocate or retire?

The AMA wrote the book—in fact, more than a dozen books—to help you with the ABCs (and even Ds!) of medical education and practice. See "Resources for a Successful Medical Career" on the next page of this brochure.

State Medical Licensure Requirements and Statistics

2007

AMA
AMERICAN
MEDICAL
ASSOCIATION

State Medical Licensure Requirements and Statistics, 2007

Internet address: www.ama-assn.org

Additional copies of this book may be ordered by calling 800 621-8335
Secure online orders can be taken at www.amabookstore.com
Mention product number OP399007

Comments or inquiries

Fred Donini-Lenhoff, Editor
Medical Education Products
American Medical Association
515 North State Street
Chicago, IL 60610
312 464-5333
312 464-5830 Fax
E-mail: fred.lenhoff@ama-assn.org
www.ama-assn.org/go/licensure

ISBN: 978-1-57947-783-7
BP15:06-P-019:8/06

Foreword

State Medical Licensure Requirements and Statistics, 2007, presents current information and statistics on medical licensure in the United States and possessions. Data were obtained from a number of sources, including state boards of medical examiners, the Federation of State Medical Boards, National Board of Medical Examiners, Educational Commission for Foreign Medical Graduates, and the United States Medical Licensing Examination Secretariat.

Licensure data and policies in this publication were compiled from the AMA's 2006 Medical Licensure Survey, which was sent in April 2006 to all 54 allopathic and 14 osteopathic boards of medical examiners in the United States. Although every effort was made to collect and record accurate data for each board, users of this book should note that the boards meet frequently and, as a result, their licensure and examination policies are modified regularly. It is therefore recommended that the state licensing boards (see Appendixes A and B) be contacted for the most up-to-date information.

In addition, boards in the following states/jurisdictions did not provide updates to the AMA in 2006 via the licensure survey:

- Oklahoma Board of Osteopathic Examiners
- Board of Medical Examiners of Puerto Rico

For more information

The AMA offers Internet information on medical licensure through its Medical Licensure Online Web site (www.ama-assn.org/go/licensure). The site includes information from this book and *Licensing and Credentialing: What Physicians Need to Know*, as well as links to state and national licensing organizations and selected articles on licensure from *American Medical News*.

Acknowledgments

The editor would like to thank the personnel of the state medical and osteopathic licensing agencies who provided statistics and licensing requirements for this publication.

Acknowledgments are also due to the following individuals and organizations for their assistance with updating copy and writing articles:

- Accreditation Council for Graduate Medical Education
  Jeanne K. Heard, MD, PhD, Director, Department of RRC Activities
  Julie Jacob, Manager of Communications
- Administrators in Medicine
  Barbara Neuman, Executive Director
- American Board of Medical Specialties
  Alexis Rodgers, Operations Manager
- Robert D. Aronson, Esq., author of "Immigration Overview for International Medical Graduates"
- Department of the Air Force
  Sharon R. Ahrari, Lieutenant Colonel, USAF, NC Chief, Credentialing and Privileging Policy
  Catherine E. Biersack, Colonel, USAF, MC Chief, Clinical Quality Management Division
- Department of the Army
  Howard M. Kimes, Colonel, US Army Director, Quality Management Directorate
  Janet L. Wilson, Lieutenant Colonel, US Army Chief, Regulatory Compliance
- Department of the Navy
  Morgan Sammons, Commander, Medical Service Corps, US Navy, Director, Clinical Operations, Bureau of Medicine and Surgery
  Georgi Irvine, Commander, Nurse Corps, US Navy (Ret), Head, Medical and Dental Staff Services, Naval Healthcare Support Office
- Drug Enforcement Administration, Office of Diversion Control
  Patricia Good, Chief, Liaison and Policy Section
- Educational Commission for Foreign Medical Graduates
  Stephen S. Seeling, JD, Vice President for Operations
  Liz Ingraham, Manager, Publications and Special Projects

- Federation of Medical Regulatory Authorities of Canada
  Fleur-Ange Lefebvre, Executive Director
- Federation of State Medical Boards of the United States
  Drew Carlson, Director of Communications
  Katherine Shelton, Communications Specialist
- Joint Commission on Accreditation of Healthcare Organizations
  Dennis O'Leary, MD, President
- National Board of Medical Examiners and United States Medical Licensing Examination Secretariat
  Kenneth E. Cotton
- National Association Medical Staff Services
  Becky Nichols, CEO
- National Committee for Quality Assurance
  L. Gregory Pawlson MD, MPH, FACP, Executive Vice President
- National Practitioner Data Bank
  Robert Oshel, MD

We would also like to acknowledge the contributions of the following AMA staff:

- Division of Survey and Data Resources
  Penny Havlicek, Monica Quiroz, Susan Montrimas, Julie Bain, Derek Smart, and Theresa Brady
- AMA Press
  Erin Vorhies, Suzanne Fraker, JD Kinney, Erica Duke, Boon Ai Tan, and Ronnie Summers
- Medical Education Products
  Enza Perrone, Dorothy Grant-Bryant, and Arecia Washington
- Continuing Physician Professional Development
  Rabia Akram
- Healthcare Education Products and Standards
  R. Mark Evans, PhD, and Patti Fitzgerald
- Project USA
  John Naughton

Fred Donini-Lenhoff, Editor

Paul H. Rockey, MD, MPH
Director, Division of Graduate Medical Education

Contents

Tables

Section I.

Licensure Policies and Regulations of State Medical/Osteopathic Boards

Administration of the United States Medical Licensing Examination Steps 1 and 2

In 1990, the Federation of State Medical Boards (FSMB) and the National Board of Medical Examiners (NBME) established the United States Medical Licensing Examination (USMLE), a single examination for assessment of US and international medical school students or graduates seeking initial licensure by US licensing jurisdictions. The USMLE replaced the Federation Licensing Examination (FLEX) and the certification examination of the NBME, as well as the Foreign Medical Graduate Examination in the Medical Sciences (FMGEMS), which was formerly used by the Educational Commission for Foreign Medical Graduates (ECFMG) for certification purposes.

The USMLE is a single examination program with three steps. Each step is complementary to the others; no step can stand alone in the assessment of readiness for medical licensure. For 2007, the fee for the Step 1 examination is $470; Step 2 CK is $470 and Step 2 CS is $1,005. Additional information on the USMLE appears on p. 80.

Thirty-one boards do not place any limits on the number of times a candidate for licensure may take USMLE Step 1; similarly, 30 boards do not place limits on taking Step 2. Twenty-three boards do not limit the amount of time in which a candidate for licensure must pass Steps 1 or 2; most of the boards with such time limits have specified a 7-year time period.

Additional Notes for Specific Licensing Jurisdictions

Texas—All candidates, except MD/PhD graduates, must pass all examination steps within 7 years. MD/PhD graduates must pass all steps within 2 years of completing the GME required for licensure in Texas. Both of these time limits may be expanded to 10 years if the applicant 1) is ABMS or AOA Bureau of Osteopathic Specialists specialty board certified, or 2) has been issued a faculty temporary license in Texas, has practiced under that permit for at least 12 months, and has been recommended for licensure by the institution at which the faculty temporary license was used.

Administration of the United States Medical Licensing Examination Step 3

(See the first two paragraphs on page 2 for general information on the USMLE.)

Many states require US or Canadian medical school graduates to have from 6 to 12 months of accredited US or Canadian graduate medical education (GME) to take USMLE Step 3. In some states, graduates of foreign medical schools are required to have completed more GME (as much as 3 years in several states). A number of states do not require completion of GME to take Step 3 or require only that a physician taking the examination be enrolled in a GME program.

Nearly all medical licensing authorities require completion of Steps 1, 2, and 3 within a 7-year period, or 10 years for those in MD/PhD or similar dual-degree programs (although 24 states may make exceptions in the event of extenuating circumstances, as noted in Table 3). Exceptions are Kansas, Maryland, and South Carolina, which allow 10 years; and California, Delaware, Florida, Louisiana, Michigan, New Hampshire, and New York, which do not impose a time limit. This 7-year period begins when the medical student or graduate first passes Step 1 or Step 2. Many licensing authorities also limit the number of attempts allowed to pass each step (particularly Step 3) and require additional education, training, or experience after a given number of failed attempts.

For 2007, the fee for the Step 3 examination is $655. Additional information on the USMLE appears on p. 80.

Additional Notes for Specific Licensing Jurisdictions

Alabama—If an applicant fails to achieve a passing score on Step 3 in three administrations, the Board may approve one additional attempt to pass Step 3 after *demonstration by the applicant of additional education, experience, or training acceptable to the Board.*

Applicants who are "dual degree candidates" (see definition, below) must achieve a passing score on Step 3 in not more than three administrations and complete Steps 1, 2, and 3 within a 10-year period, beginning when the applicant initially passes his or her first step. The Board does not accept scores from a retaking of a previously passed step of the USMLE.

For purposes of the USMLE, dual degree candidates are defined as the following:

- The applicant is pursuing the MD or DO degree and the PhD degree in an institution or program accredited by the LCME and a regional university accrediting body; and
- The applicant is a student in good standing, enrolled in the institution or program; and
- The PhD studies are in a field of biological sciences tested in the USMLE Step 1 content, including, but not limited to, anatomy, biochemistry, physiology, microbiology, pharmacology, pathology, genetics, neuroscience, and molecular biology.

Arizona—No time limit for USMLE Step 3 for applicants who hold a license in another jurisdiction (licensure by endorsement); for initial licensure, the 7-year limit applies.

Ohio—All 3 steps must have been passed within a 7-year period, and the performance achieved on each step must have been recognized by the USMLE as a recommended passing performance. A limited exception to this rule may be granted to an applicant who in conjunction with a medical degree is actively pursuing a doctoral degree in an institution or program accredited by the Liaison Committee on Medical Education and a regional university accrediting body. The applicant must be a student in good standing when enrolled in the institution or program, and the doctoral degree must be in a field of biological sciences tested in the Step 1 content. These fields include, but are not necessarily limited to, anatomy, biochemistry, physiology, microbiology, pharmacology, genetics, neuroscience, and molecular biology. Fields not excepted include, but are not necessarily limited to, business, economics, ethics, history, and other fields not directly related to biological science. A limited exception to this rule may also be granted to an applicant who suffered from a significant health condition which by its severity would necessarily cause a delay to the applicant's medical study. Regardless, all three steps must have been passed within a 10-year period.

Oregon—A waiver is allowed of the three attempt limit for USMLE Step 3 (1 year approved GME after third failed attempt before fourth and final attempt) for applicants who are ABMS certified.

A waiver of the 7-year time limit for completion of USMLE Steps 1, 2, and 3 is allowed for applicants who are ABMS certified, have participated in a combined MD/PhD or DO/PhD program, suffered from a documented significant health condition that by its severity would necessarily cause delay to an applicant's medical study, or have completed continuous GME equivalent to an MD/PhD or DO/PhD program.

Texas—All candidates, except MD/PhD graduates, must pass all examination steps within 7 years. MD/PhD graduates must pass all steps within 2 years of completing the GME required for licensure in Texas. Both of these time limits may be expanded to 10 years if the applicant 1) is ABMS or AOA Bureau of Osteopathic Specialists specialty board certified, or 2) has been issued a faculty temporary license in Texas, has practiced under that permit for at least 12 months, and has been recommended for licensure by the institution at which the faculty temporary license was used.

Virgin Islands—The USMLE is not administered; SPEX is used to evaluate physicians' knowledge.

Table 1
Administration of the US Medical Licensing Examination Steps 1 and 2

	Number of Times Candidates for Licensure May Take USMLE Step 1	Number of Times Candidates for Licensure May Take USMLE Step 2	Amount of Time Within Which Steps 1 and 2 of USMLE Must Be Passed
Alabama	No limit	No limit	No limit
Alaska	1	1	7 yrs
Arizona	No limit	No limit	No limit
Arkansas	6	6	7 yrs
California	No limit	No limit	No limit
Colorado	No limit	No limit	No limit
Connecticut	No limit	No limit	No limit
Delaware	No limit	No limit	No limit
DC	No limit	No limit	No limit
Florida	No limit	No limit	No limit
Georgia	No limit	No limit	7 yrs (9 yrs for MD/PhD programs)
Guam	Not applicable	Not applicable	Not applicable
Hawaii	No limit	No limit	No limit
Idaho	2	2	No limit
Illinois	5	5	7 yrs
Indiana	5	5	7 yrs (all 3 steps)
Iowa	6	6	7 yrs (all 3 steps)
Kansas	No limit	No limit	10 yrs (all 3 steps)
Kentucky	No limit	No limit	No limit
Louisiana	No limit	4	No limit
Maine	No limit	No limit	7 yrs (all 3 steps)
Maryland	4	4	No limit
Massachusetts	No limit	No limit	7 yrs (all 3 steps)
Michigan	No limit	No limit	No limit
Minnesota	3	3	7 yrs (all 3 steps)
Mississippi	No limit	No limit	No limit
Missouri	3	3	7 yrs (all 3 steps)
Montana	No limit	No limit	No limit
Nebraska	4	4	7 yrs (all 3 steps)
Nevada	No limit	No limit	7 yrs (all 3 steps and 9 total attempts)
New Hampshire	3	3	No limit
New Jersey	No limit	No limit	7 yrs
New Mexico	6	6	7 yrs (all 3 steps)
New York	No limit	No limit	No limit
North Carolina	6	6	7 yrs (all 3 steps); 10 yrs for MD/PhDs
North Dakota	3	3	7 yrs (all 3 steps)

(continued on next page)

Table 1 (continued)
Administration of the US Medical Licensing Examination Steps 1 and 2

	Number of Times Candidates for Licensure May Take USMLE Step 1	Number of Times Candidates for Licensure May Take USMLE Step 2	Amount of Time Within Which Steps 1 and 2 of USMLE Must Be Passed
Ohio	No limit	No limit	7 yrs
Oklahoma	3	3	7 yrs (all 3 steps)
Oregon	No limit	No limit	7 yrs (all 3 steps)
Pennsylvania	No limit	No limit	No limit
Puerto Rico	No limit	No limit	7 yrs
Rhode Island	3	3	7 yrs
South Carolina	4	4	10 yrs (all 3 steps)
South Dakota	3	3	7 yrs (all 3 steps)
Tennessee	No limit	No limit	No limit
Texas*	3	3	7 yrs (all 3 steps); 10 yrs for MD/PhDs
Utah	3	3	7 yrs (10 yrs for MD/PhD programs)
Vermont	No limit	No limit	7 yrs
Virgin Islands	Not applicable	Not applicable	Not applicable
Virginia	No limit	No limit	No limit
Washington	No limit	No limit	No limit
West Virginia	No limit	No limit	7 yrs
Wisconsin	3	3	7 yrs
Wyoming	No limit	No limit	No limit (subject to Board discretion)

* Refer to introductory text to this table for more information on this state's regulations.

Note: ***All information should be verified with the licensing board; licenses based on endorsement are granted to those physicians meeting all state requirements.***

Table 2
Administration of the US Medical Licensing Examination Step 3: Graduate Medical Education Requirements

	Amount of Accredited US or Canadian GME Required to Take USMLE Step 3	
	Graduates of US/Canadian Medical Schools	Graduates of Foreign Medical Schools
Alabama	None (but must be enrolled in GME prgm)	2 yrs (must be enrolled in third yr of GME prgm)
Alaska	1 yr	1 yr
Arizona	6 mos	6 mos
Arkansas	None	None
California	None	None
Colorado	1 yr	3 yrs
Connecticut	None	None
Delaware	1 yr	1 yr
DC	1 yr	3 yrs
Florida	None	None
Georgia	1 yr	1-3 yrs
Guam	2 yrs	2 yrs
Hawaii	None (must be enrolled in first yr of GME prgm)	1 yr (and must be enrolled in second year of GME prgm)
Idaho	9 mos	2 yrs, 9 mos
Illinois	1 yr	1 yr
Indiana	6 mos	2 yrs
Iowa	7 mos (or enrollment in approved GME program)	7 mos (or enrollment in approved GME program)
Kansas	1 yr (or enrollment in GME program in Kansas)	3 yrs (2 in US) (or enrollment in GME program in Kansas)
Kentucky	1 yr	1 yr
Louisiana	None	None
Maine	1 yr	2 yrs (plus ECFMG certificate)
Maryland	None	None
Massachusetts	1 yr	1 yr
Michigan	6 mos	6 mos
Minnesota	None (but must be enrolled in GME prgm)	None (but must be enrolled in GME prgm)
Mississippi	1 yr	3 yrs
Missouri	1 yr	3 yrs
Montana	2 yrs	3 yrs
Nebraska	None	None
Nevada	None	None
New Hampshire	1 yr	1 yr
New Jersey	1 yr	1 yr
New Mexico	1 yr	1 yr
New York	None	None
North Carolina	None	3 yrs (none if enrolled in GME pgm in state)
North Dakota	6 mos	1 yr
Ohio	9 mos	9 mos
Oklahoma	None	None

(continued on next page)

Table 2 (continued)
Administration of the US Medical Licensing Examination Step 3: Graduate Medical Education Requirements

	Amount of Accredited US or Canadian GME Required to Take USMLE Step 3	
	Graduates of US/Canadian Medical Schools	Graduates of Foreign Medical Schools
Oregon	None (but must be enrolled in GME prgm)	None (but must be enrolled in GME prgm)
Pennsylvania	None (but must be enrolled in GME prgm)	None (but must be enrolled in GME prgm)
Puerto Rico	None	None
Rhode Island	1 yr	1 yr
South Carolina	1 yr	3 yrs
South Dakota	None	1 yr
Tennessee	1 yr	1 yr
Texas	None	None
Utah	None	None (must be ECFMG-certified)
Vermont	7 mos	7 mos
Virgin Islands	Not applicable	Not applicable
Virginia	None	None
Washington	1 yr (or enrolled in GME program)	1 yr (or enrolled in GME program)
West Virginia	None	None
Wisconsin	1 yr	1 yr
Wyoming	1 yr	2 yrs (subject to Board discretion)

Abbreviations

USMLE—United States Medical Licensing Examination
ECFMG—Educational Commission for Foreign Medical Graduates
GME—graduate medical education

Note: ***All information should be verified with the licensing board; medical licenses are granted to those physicians meeting all state requirements—at the discretion of the board.***

Table 3
Administration of the US Medical Licensing Examination Step 3: Time Limits for Completion

	Number of Times Candidates for Licensure May Take USMLE Step 3	Requirements to Repeat Step 3 if Not Passed in Designated Number of Attempts	Time Limit for Completion of All Steps of USMLE	Time Limit for MD/PhD or Dual-Degree Candidates	Time Limit May be Waived in Event of Extenuating Circumstances
Alabama*	3	Further education, training, or experience	7 yrs	10 yrs	No
Alaska	1		7 yrs		No
Arizona*	No limit		7 yrs (initial applicants only)		No
Arkansas	6		7 yrs		
California	No limit		No limit		—
Colorado	No limit		7 yrs	10 yrs	Yes
Connecticut	No limit		7 yrs		No
Delaware	No limit		No limit		No
DC	No limit	After 3 failed attempts, 1 additional yr ACGME- or AOA-approved GME	7 yrs		Yes
Florida	No limit		No limit		—
Georgia	3	1 yr of additional Board-approved training	7 yrs	9 yrs	Yes
Guam	No limit		7 yrs		No
Hawaii	No limit		7 yrs		No
Idaho	2	Remedial training	7 yrs	10 yrs	Yes
Illinois	5	Further education, experience, or remedial training	7 yrs		Yes
Indiana	5		7 yrs		No
Iowa	3	After 3 failed attempts, 3 yrs of progressive GME required	7 yrs (If not passed within 7 yrs, ABMS or AOA board certification required)	10 yrs	Yes
Kansas	3	After 3 failed attempts, further education, training, or experience	10 yrs		No
Kentucky	No limit		7 yrs		Yes
Louisiana	4	After 3 failed attempts, 6 mos of additional GME	No limit		—
Maine	3		7 yrs		Yes
Maryland	4	After 3 failed attempts, 1 yr additional GME; no more than 3 failures permitted on any 1 step	10 yrs		Yes
Massachusetts	6		7 yrs		Yes
Michigan	No limit	After 5 yrs from first attempt, additional GME in Board-approved program in-state	No limit		—
Minnesota	3		7 yrs	7 yrs plus time to obtain non-MD degree, or 10 yrs, whichever comes first	
Mississippi	3	After 3 failed attempts, 1 additional yr ACGME- or AOA-approved GME	7 yrs		Yes
Missouri	3		7 yrs		No
Montana	3		7 yrs		Yes

(continued on next page)

Table 3 (continued)
Administration of the US Medical Licensing Examination Step 3: Time Limits for Completion

	Number of Times Candidates for Licensure May Take USMLE Step 3	Requirements to Repeat Step 3 if Not Passed in Designated Number of Attempts	Amount of Time Within Which All Steps of USMLE Must Be Passed	Time Limit for MD/PhD or Dual-Degree Candidates	Time Limit May be Waived in Event of Extenuating Circumstances
Nebraska	4		7 yrs		No
Nevada	No limit		7 yrs (all 3 steps and 9 total attempts)		Yes
New Hampshire	3	Further education, training, or experience	No limit		—
New Jersey	5	Further education, training, or experience	7 yrs (if not passed, must repeat entire sequence)		Yes
New Mexico	6 (within 7 yrs of first pass)		7 yrs		Yes
New York	No limit		No limit		—
North Carolina	6		7 yrs	10 yrs	Yes
North Dakota	3		7 yrs		Yes
Ohio*	No limit		7 yrs	10 yrs	Yes
Oklahoma	3		7 yrs	10 yrs (pending)	No
Oregon	4	After 3 failed attempts, 1 yr of GME required before 4th attempt	7 yrs	10 yrs	Yes
Pennsylvania	No limit	After 3 failed attempts, further education required	7 yrs		Yes
Puerto Rico	No limit		7 yrs		
Rhode Island	3		7 yrs		Yes
South Carolina	4		10 yrs		No
South Dakota	3		7 yrs (Board may grant exceptions if candidate is Board-certified)		No
Tennessee	No limit		7 yrs		No
Texas*	3		7 yrs	10 yrs	No
Utah	3	Remedial training	7 yrs	10 yrs	No
Vermont	3		7 yrs		No
Virgin Islands*	Not applicable		Not applicable		No
Virginia	3		7 yrs (Board may grant exceptions for good cause)		Yes
Washington	3	Remedial training	7 yrs	10 yrs	Yes
West Virginia	No limit		7 yrs	10 yrs	No
Wisconsin	3		7 yrs		No
Wyoming	2	1 additional yr of ACGME-accredited GME	7 yrs		Yes

Abbreviations
ACGME—Accreditation Council for Graduate Medical Education
AOA—American Osteopathic Association
USMLE—United States Medical Licensing Examination
ECFMG—Educational Commission for Foreign Medical Graduates
GME—graduate medical education

* Refer to introductory text to this table for more information on this state's regulations.

Note: ***All information should be verified with the licensing board; medical licenses are granted to those physicians meeting all state requirements—at the discretion of the board.***

Endorsement Policies for Physicians Holding an Initial License

Endorsement is the process through which a state issues an unrestricted license to practice medicine to an individual who holds a valid and unrestricted license in another jurisdiction. Licensure endorsement, previously referred to as "reciprocity," is generally based on documentation of successfully completing approved examinations, authentication of required core documents, and completion of any additional requirements assessing the applicant's fitness to practice medicine in the new jurisdiction. Each state has strict endorsement requirements.

Policies of medical/osteopathic licensing boards for endorsement of medical/osteopathic licensing examinations taken before and after the development of the Federation Licensing Examination (FLEX) vary from state to state. Each state board created its own licensing examination before FLEX, which may partially explain the sizable variation in endorsement policies from one state to another. Some boards will endorse scores on state licensing examinations in use prior to the development of FLEX; these scores may be endorsed in connection with a passing score on the Special Purpose Examination (SPEX). Endorsement of a certificate of the National Board of Medical Examiners (NBME) or of an examination refers to issuance of a license based on an acceptable score on the NBME or the state's board exam.

Forty-four state medical boards require some or all candidates for licensure endorsement to appear for an interview; six boards require some or all candidates to appear for an oral examination.

Fourteen boards require that a license be endorsed within a certain period after examination (usually 10 years). In most of these 14 states, SPEX is required if the time limit is not met.

All medical boards will accept or consider for endorsement the national board certificate of the NBME or the United States Medical Licensing Examination (USMLE), except the Virgin Islands, which does not accept endorsements. A number of osteopathic boards do not accept USMLE for licensure by endorsement.

Forty-seven boards will endorse the Licentiate of the Medical Council of Canada (LMCC); 35 will endorse the certificates of the National Board of Osteopathic Medical Examiners (NBOME); 29 will endorse a state board examination (designated "SBE" in Table 4) from another jurisdiction, occasionally in combination with a certificate from an American Board of Medical Specialties (ABMS) specialty board; nine will endorse the Comprehensive Osteopathic Medical Licensing Examination (COMLEX) of the NBOME; four will endorse FLEX; and three will endorse an ABMS board certificate. (Endorsement of these credentials is subject to any specific requirements in effect in that state.)

Additional Notes for Specific Licensing Jurisdictions

Colorado—LMCC is accepted or considered for endorsement for graduates of US or Canadian medical schools only.

Connecticut—Before June 1985: 75 on day 3 of FLEX to combine best scores (within 7 years); FWA truncated.

Idaho—FLEX scores obtained at different sittings cannot be combined. Applicants who fail to pass the FLEX or USMLE on two separate occasions will not be eligible to take the examination for at least 1 year, and before taking either examination again, they must show the board that they have successfully engaged in a course of study to improve their ability to engage in the practice of medicine.

LMCC is endorsed only for graduates of US or Canadian medical schools.

Illinois—Applicant had to pass all three parts of the pre-1985 FLEX in the same state.

Iowa—Applicants who took old (pre-1985) FLEX must provide evidence of at least two of the following: (1) certification under seal that the applicant passed FLEX with a FLEX-weighted average of 75% or better, as determined by the state medical licensing authority, in no more than two sittings; (2) verification under seal of medical licensure in the state that administered the examination; (3) evidence of current certification by an American specialty board approved or recognized by the Council of Medical Education of the AMA or the ABMS or AOA.

Louisiana—At board discretion, candidates for licensure endorsement must appear.

SPEX may be waived if an applicant was certified or recertified by an ABMS board within 10 years of the application date.

Maryland—SPEX is required if active licensure was interrupted during the last 10 years and if physician has not passed a written licensure exam within the last 15 years and has neither ABMS lifetime or time-limited certification.

Minnesota—SPEX may be waived if the applicant is currently certified by an ABMS board, an AOA specialty board, or a Canadian specialty board.

Mississippi—FLEX scores obtained at different sittings cannot be combined. An exemption may be granted to the weighted average of 75 on FLEX if the applicant has completed an approved GME program and is ABMS or AOA board certified.

LMCC is accepted or considered for endorsement for graduates of US or Canadian medical schools only.

SPEX may be waived if an applicant was certified or recertified by an ABMS board within 10 years of the application date.

North Carolina—Licensure by endorsement requires a valid and unrestricted license to practice medicine in another state based on an examination testing general medical knowledge, or passing of a licensure examination testing general medical knowledge that is determined by the board as equivalent to the board's examination.

Oregon—SPEX may be waived if an applicant was 1) ABMS certified or recertified within 10 years of date of applying for an Oregon license, or 2) completed an accredited 1-year residency or a board-approved clinical fellowship, or 3) obtained CME to the Board's satisfaction.

Texas—All candidates for licensure must appear, present original documents for inspection, and pass the Texas Medical Jurisprudence Examination.

Candidates who have not been examined for licensure in the preceding 10-year period prior to filing their application must pass the SPEX;

-or- have passed a specialty certification/recertification examination or formal evaluation or an examination of continued demonstration of qualifications by an ABMS or Bureau of Osteopathic Specialist member board within the preceding 10 years;

-or- have obtained, through extraordinary circumstances, unique training equal to the training required for specialty certification as determined by a committee of the board and approved by the board.

SPEX may be waived if an applicant was certified or recertified by an ABMS board within 10 years of the application date.

Utah—LMCC is accepted or considered for endorsement for graduates of US or Canadian medical schools only.

Table 4
Endorsement Policies for Physicians Holding an Initial License

	Requirements for Endorsement of License Based on FLEX			Requirements for Candidates' Appearance			Maximum Time for Licensure Endorsement After Examination		Credential Also Accepted or Considered for Endorsement (in Addition to USMLE and NBME)
	Exceptions to 75 FWA on 3-part FLEX	Must Pass 3-Part (Pre-1985) FLEX in One Sitting	Must Pass 2-Part (1985-93) FLEX in One Sitting	Candidates Who Must Appear...	...for Oral Exam	...for Interview	Time	Additional Requirements if Time Limit Not Met	
Alabama	None	No	No	Some			10 yrs	SPEX, ABMS	LMCC
Alaska	None	No	No	Some		X	None		LMCC, NBOME
Arizona	None	Yes	No	Some		X	10 yrs	SPEX, ABMS	LMCC
Arizona DO	None	No	No	Some	X	X	7 yrs		SBE (pre-FLEX), NBOME
Arkansas	None	Yes	No	IMGs		X	None		LMCC
California	None	Yes	No	None			None		LMCC
California DO	None	No	No	None					NBOME
Colorado*	None	Yes	No	None			None		LMCC
Connecticut*	*See note*	No	No	None			None		LMCC, SBE, NBOME
Delaware	None	No	No	All		X	None		LMCC
DC	None	Yes	No	None			None		LMCC, NBOME
Florida	None	Yes	No	Some		X	None		
Florida DO	NA	NA	NA	Some		X	None		SBE, NBOME, COMVEX
Georgia	None	Yes	No	Some		X	None		LMCC, SBE, NBOME, COMLEX
Guam	None	Yes	Yes	Some		X	10 yrs	SPEX	NBOME
Hawaii	None	No	No	None			None		
Hawaii DO	None	No	No	None			None		NBOME
Idaho*	*See note*	Yes	No	Some		X	5 yrs	SPEX	LMCC, SBE, NBOME
Illinois*	None	No	No	Some		X	None		LMCC, NBOME
Indiana	Split scores okay	No	No	Some		X	None		LMCC
Iowa*	*See note*	No	No	Some		X	None		LMCC, SBE, NBOME
Kansas	None	Yes	No	Some		X	None		LMCC, SBE (pre-'72) NBOME, COMLEX
Kentucky	None	Yes	No	Some			None		LMCC, NBOME
Louisiana*	None	Yes	No	Some		X	10 yrs	SPEX	SBE
Maine	None	No	No	Some		X	None		LMCC, SBE, GMC
Maine DO	None	No	No	Some		X	None	SPEX	NBOME
Maryland*	None	Yes	No	None			15 yrs	SPEX	LMCC, NBOME
Massachusetts	None	Yes	Yes	Some		X	None	Current evaluations	LMCC, NBOME, COMLEX
Michigan	None	Yes	No	None			None		LMCC, SBE
Michigan DO	NA	NA	NA	None					NBOME, SBE (pre-FLEX)
Minnesota*	None	Yes (5 tries)	No (3 tries)	All		X	10 yrs	SPEX, ABMS	LMCC, SBE, NBOME, COMLEX
Mississippi*	*See note*	Yes	No	All		X	10 yrs	SPEX, ABMS	LMCC, SBE (pre-1973), NBOME
Missouri	None	Yes	No	Some		X	None		LMCC, NBOME
Montana	None	No	No	Some		X	None		LMCC

(continued on next page)

Table 4 (continued)
Endorsement Policies for Physicians Holding an Initial License

	Requirements for Endorsement of License Based on FLEX			Requirements for Candidates' Appearance			Maximum Time for Licensure Endorsement After Examination		Credential Also Accepted or Considered for Endorsement (in Addition to USMLE and NBME)
	Exceptions to 75 FWA on 3-part FLEX	Must Pass 3-Part (Pre-1985) FLEX in One Sitting	Must Pass 2-Part (1985-92) FLEX in One Sitting	Candidates Who Must Appear...	...for Oral Exam	...for Interview	Time	Additional Requirements if Time Limit Not Met	
Nebraska	None	Yes	No	None			None		LMCC, SBE
Nevada	None	No	No	All		X	None		LMCC
Nevada DO	None	No	No	None			10 yrs	ABMS exam, COMVEX, SPEX	SBE (pre-FLEX) NBOME
New Hampshire	None	No	No	None			None	May require exam, interview, proof of clinical competence, etc	LMCC, SBE
New Jersey	Pre-Jan 1981: 74.5 FWA	No	No	Some		X	None		LMCC w/ABMS & SBE; ABMS w/SBE
New Mexico	None	No	No	Some		X	None		LMCC, SBE, FLEX (pre-1974)
New Mexico DO	None	No	No	All		X			NBOME, FLEX, COMLEX
New York	None	No; 5-year period to pass all parts	No; 5-year period to pass all parts	None			None		LMCC (with a valid Canadian provincial license), ABMS, foreign license
North Carolina	None	No	No	Some	Some	Some	10 yrs	Training, SPEX, AMA PRA, ABMS	SBE, FLEX, COMLEX
North Dakota	None	Yes	No	Some		X	None		LMCC, SBE, NBOME, COMLEX
Ohio	72 if taken during first 2 yrs of a state's administration and accepted as passing by state	Yes	No	None			None		LMCC (professional experience in US or abroad)
Oklahoma	None	Yes	No	Some		X	None		LMCC
Oklahoma DO	NA			Some		X			NBOME
Oregon*	None	Yes	No	Some		X	7 yrs	SPEX	LMCC, NBOME, SBE, FLEX, COMLEX
Pennsylvania	None	No	No	None			None		LMCC
Pennsylvania DO	None	No	No	None			None		SBE, NBOME
Puerto Rico	None	Yes	Yes	None			None		
Rhode Island	None	No	No	Some		X	None		LMCC, NBOME
South Carolina	None	Yes	No	All		X	10 yrs	SPEX	LMCC, SBE w/ABMS, NBOME
South Dakota	None	Yes	Yes	Some		X	None		LMCC
Tennessee	None	Yes	Yes	Some		X	None		LMCC, ABMS
Tennessee DO	None	No	No	Some	X	X			NBOME
Texas*	None	Yes	No	All		X	10 yrs	SPEX	LMCC, NBOME, COMLEX
Utah	None	No	No	Some		X	None	Retake exams	LMCC, SBE
Vermont	None	Yes	Yes	All		X	None		LMCC, ABMS
Vermont DO	None	No	No	None					SBE (pre-FLEX), NBOME

Table 4 (continued)
Endorsement Policies for Physicians Holding an Initial License

	Requirements for Endorsement of License Based on FLEX			Requirements for Candidates' Appearance			Maximum Time for Licensure Endorsement After Examination		Credential Also Accepted or Considered for Endorsement (in Addition to USMLE and NBME)
	Exceptions to 75 FWA on 3-part FLEX	Must Pass 3-Part (Pre-1985) FLEX in One Sitting	Must Pass 2-Part (1985-92) FLEX in One Sitting	Candidates Who Must Appear...	...for Oral Exam	...for Interview	Time	Additional Requirements if Time Limit Not Met	
Virgin Islands	**No reciprocity or endorsement; all licensure candidates must sit for complete SPEX exam.**								
Virginia	None	No (unless taken pre-June 1976)	Yes	Some		X	None		LMCC, pre-1970=SBE, with ABMS
Washington	None	No	No	None			None		LMCC (post-1969)
Washington DO	None	No	No	None					SBE (pre-FLEX), NBOME
West Virginia	None	Yes	No	All		X	None		LMCC, SBE
West Virginia DO	NA	NA	NA	All		X			SBE (pre-FLEX) NBOME
Wisconsin	None	Yes	No	Some	X	X	None		LMCC (post-1978)
Wyoming	None	Yes	No	All	X	X	None		LMCC, SBE, NBOME

Abbreviations

FWA—Federation Licensing Examination (FLEX) Weighted Average, which applied to the pre-1985 three-part FLEX and gave greater weight to parts 2 and 3; all states currently require a minimum passing score of 75 on each component of the post-1985 two-part FLEX.

ABMS—certification from a member board of the American Board of Medical Specialties

COMLEX—Comprehensive Osteopathic Medical Licensing Examination

COMVEX—Comprehensive Osteopathic Medical Variable Purpose Examination

FLEX—Federation Licensing Examination

GMC—General Medical Council of the United Kingdom

IMG—international medical graduate

LMCC—certification by the Licentiate of the Medical Council of Canada

NBME—certificate of the National Board of Medical Examiners

NBOME—certificate from the National Board of Osteopathic Medical Examiners

SBE—state board examination

SPEX—Special Purpose Examination

USMLE—United States Medical Licensing Examination

* Refer to introductory text to this table for more information on this state's regulations.

Note: ***All information should be verified with the licensing board; licenses based on endorsement are granted to those physicians meeting all state requirements.***

Additional Requirements for Endorsement of Licenses Held by International Medical Graduates

In all states, international medical graduates (IMGs) seeking licensure by endorsement must meet the same requirements as US graduates (listed in Table 4), in addition to the requirements in Table 5.

All states except California and West Virginia require that IMGs seeking licensure endorsement hold a certificate from the Educational Commission for Foreign Medical Graduates (ECFMG). In lieu of holding that certificate, a candidate for licensure in North Dakota may have passed a certification examination of an American Board of Medical Specialties (ABMS) board.

About half of the boards require IMG candidates to have graduated from a state-approved foreign medical school; several boards also maintain and use a list of approved/unapproved foreign medical schools for decisions on initial licensure (see Table 9, column 3). A number of boards require 3 years of US or Canadian GME, and a majority of jurisdictions also may require an interview or oral examination prior to endorsement.

Note: Physicians who graduated via the Fifth Pathway are not required to have an ECFMG certificate. For more information on the Fifth Pathway, see p. 28.

Additional Notes for Specific Licensing Jurisdictions

California—Four years' licensure required for IMGs, in addition to 2 years of ACGME-accredited training (or 1 year of ACGME-accredited training plus ABMS, or 1 year of ACGME-accredited training plus SPEX).

Connecticut—State-approved foreign medical school must have been listed with the World Health Organization in 1970 (or by individual review).

Florida—Rules on clinical clerkships for IMGs adopted by the Florida Board before October 1986 do not apply to any graduate who had already completed a clinical clerkship or who had begun a clinical clerkship, as long as the clerkship was completed within 3 years.

Illinois—Candidate must have completed a 6-year postsecondary course of study, comprising 2 academic years of liberal arts instruction, 2 academic years in basic sciences, and 2 academic years in clinical sciences, while enrolled in the medical school that confirmed the degree.

Iowa—Requirement for graduation from a state-approved medical school is waived if candidate passed the Special Purpose Examination (SPEX) or state science examination, or completed 3 years of GME in an ACGME-accredited residency program, or held a permanent license to practice without restrictions in a US jurisdiction for at least 5 years.

Two years of accredited US or Canadian GME is required as of July 1, 2006.

Maryland—In addition to 2 years of ACGME- or AOA-accredited GME, 1 year of GME required if candidate failed any part of an examination three times; no more than three failures permitted.

Minnesota—SPEX is required if candidate took initial licensing exam more than 10 years ago, unless candidate is currently ABMS/AOA or Canadian medical specialty board certified.

North Dakota—The ECFMG certificate requirement is waived for holders of the Fifth Pathway and for graduates of medical schools in Canada, England, Scotland, Ireland, Australia, or New Zealand. The requirement may be waived, by unanimous vote of the Board, for holders of ABMS certification.

The requirement for 3 years of US/Canadian GME is waived if the candidate holds an ABMS board certificate or has passed SPEX and (a) has successfully completed 1 year of state-approved GME in the US or Canada (or 3 years of GME in the United Kingdom), (b) has other professional experience and training equivalent to GME years 2 and 3, and (c) meets all other licensing requirements.

Oregon—Candidate must have attended a foreign school listed with the WHO that is chartered in the country in which it is located and provides four full terms of instruction of 8 months of physical on-site attendance of courses in the country in which the school is chartered. This requirement may be waived for ABMS certified candidates who substantially met attendance requirements.

Rhode Island—Candidate must have obtained supervised clinical training in the US as part of the medical school curriculum in a hospital affiliated with an LCME-accredited medical school or an ACGME-accredited residency.

Texas—All IMG candidates for licensure must appear for interview, present original documents for inspection, and pass the Texas Medical Jurisprudence Examination.

Table 5
Additional Requirements for Endorsement of Licenses Held by International Medical Graduates
IMGs must also meet all the requirements for endorsement listed in Table 4

	Must Have ECFMG Certificate	Must Have Graduated From State-approved Foreign Medical School *(cf Table 9, Column 3)*	Must Appear for…		Amount of Accredited US or Canadian GME Required	Notes
			Interview	Possible Interview		
Alabama	Yes	Yes				SPEX (if no ABMS or SBE within 10 yrs)
Alaska	Yes	No		Yes		
Arizona	Yes	No				SPEX if exam is over 10 yrs (and no current ABMS)
Arkansas	Yes	Yes	Yes		3 yrs	
California*	No	Yes				
Colorado	Yes	Yes				
Connecticut*	Yes	Yes				
Delaware	Yes	No	Yes			
DC	Yes	Yes				
Florida*	Yes	No		Yes	2 yrs	
Georgia	Yes	Yes		Yes	3 yrs	
Guam	Yes	No		Yes		
Hawaii	Yes	No				
Idaho	Yes	Yes		Yes	3 yrs	Unapproved medical school graduates must meet additional requirements
Illinois*	Yes	No		Yes	2 yrs	
Indiana	Yes	Yes		Yes	2 yrs	
Iowa*	Yes	No		Yes	2 yrs	
Kansas	Yes	No		Yes	2 yrs	Foreign med school must have been in existence 15 yrs
Kentucky	Yes	Yes		Yes	2 yrs	
Louisiana	Yes	Yes	Yes		3 yrs	
Maine	Yes	Yes		Yes	3 yrs	Foreign medical school must be listed with ECFMG
Maryland*	Yes	No			2 yrs	
Massachusetts	Yes	No		Yes	2 yrs	
Michigan	Yes	No			2 yrs	
Minnesota*	Yes	Yes	Yes		2 yrs	SPEX is required
Mississippi	Yes	Yes	Yes		3 yrs	
Missouri	Yes	Yes		Yes	3 yrs	
Montana	Yes	Yes		Yes	3 yrs	
Nebraska	Yes	No			3 yrs	
Nevada	Yes	No		Yes	3 yrs	SPEX (if no ABMS or NBME/FLEX/USMLE within 10 yrs)
New Hampshire	Yes	No				
New Jersey	Yes	No		Yes		
New Mexico	Yes	Yes		Yes		Must be board-certified in ABMS-recognized specialty
New York	Yes	No				
North Carolina	Yes	No		Yes	3 yrs	
North Dakota*	Yes	Yes		Yes	3 yrs	
Ohio	Yes	No			2 yrs	

(continued on next page)

Table 5 (continued)
Additional Requirements for Endorsement of Licenses Held by International Medical Graduates
IMGs must also meet all the requirements for endorsement listed in Table 4

	Must Have ECFMG Certificate	Must Have Graduated From State-approved Foreign Medical School *(cf Table 9, Column 3)*	Must Appear for...		Amount of Accredited US or Canadian GME Required	Notes
			Interview	Possible Interview		
Oklahoma	Yes	Yes			2 yrs	
Oregon	Yes	Yes		Yes	3 yrs	Foreign medical school must be listed with ECFMG
Pennsylvania	Yes	No		Yes	3 yrs	Foreign medical school must be listed with ECFMG
Puerto Rico	Yes	Yes				
Rhode Island*	Yes	Yes		Yes	3 yrs	1 yr of advanced standing recognized if granted by ABMS
South Carolina	Yes	No	Yes		3 yrs	For Fifth Pathway candidates, ABMS/AOA cert. required
South Dakota	Yes	Yes		Yes		
Tennessee	Yes	Yes		Yes		
Texas*	Yes	No	Yes		3 yrs	
Utah	Yes	No		Yes	2 yrs	
Vermont	Yes	Yes	Yes		3 yrs	
Virginia	Yes	No		Yes	2 yrs	Licensure in another state can replace ECFMG cert.
Washington	Yes	No			2 yrs	
West Virginia	No	No	Yes		3 yrs	3 yrs GME, or 1 yr plus ABMS certification
Wisconsin	Yes	No				Possible oral exam
Wyoming	Yes	No			2 yrs	

Abbreviations

ABMS—American Board of Medical Specialties
ECFMG—Educational Commission for Foreign Medical Graduates
FMGEMS—Foreign Medical Graduate Examination in the Medical Sciences
IMG—international medical graduate
SBE—state board examination
SPEX—Special Purpose Examination
VQE—Visa Qualifying Examination

* Refer to introductory text to this table for more information on this state's regulations.

Note: ***All information should be verified with the licensing board; licenses based on endorsement are granted to those physicians meeting all state requirements.***

Policies About the Special Purpose Examination (SPEX)

The Special Purpose Examination (SPEX), a 1-day, computer-administered examination with approximately 420 multiple-choice questions, assesses knowledge required of all physicians, regardless of specialty. SPEX is used to assess physicians who have held a valid, unrestricted license in a US or Canadian jurisdiction who are:

A. Required by the state medical board to demonstrate current medical knowledge,

B. Seeking endorsement licensure some years beyond initial examination, or

C. Seeking license reinstatement after a period of professional inactivity. Physicians holding a valid, unrestricted license may also apply for SPEX, independent of any request or approval from a medical licensing board.

For more information on SPEX, see p. 90.

Fifty-five jurisdictions use SPEX to assess current competence or if a candidate has not taken a written licensure exam or the American Board of Medical Specialties (ABMS) board certification examination within a specified number of years (usually 10). In 27 jurisdictions, SPEX scores are valid for an unlimited length of time. Forty-three jurisdictions will accept SPEX scores from other licensing jurisdictions.

Additional Notes for Specific Licensing Jurisdictions

Florida—SPEX is offered only to candidates who have actively practiced medicine for at least 10 years after obtaining a valid license in a jurisdiction or a combination of jurisdictions in the United States or Canada and who meet Florida's licensure requirements.

Maryland—SPEX is required if active licensure was interrupted during the last 10 years and if a physician has not passed a written licensure examination within the last 15 years and an ABMS board certification examination within the last 10 years.

North Dakota—SPEX (or ABMS board certification) is required when a candidate is being considered for the following exception: If the candidate has not completed 3 years of GME but has met all other licensing requirements and has successfully completed 1 year of US or Canadian GME in a board-approved program, and if the board finds that the candidate has other professional experience and training substantially equivalent to the second and third years of GME, then the candidate may be eligible for licensure.

Texas—SPEX scores accepted from other licensing jurisdictions if a candidate passed with a score of 75 or higher.

Vermont DO—SPEX or COMVEX (Comprehensive Osteopathic Medical Variable purpose Examination), or both, may be required to reinstate an expired license.

West Virginia DO—COMVEX may be required.

Table 6
Policies About the Special Purpose Examination

	SPEX May Be Required...	...for the Following Reasons	...to Assess Current Competence	...if Written Licensure Exam or ABMS Certification Exam Has Not Been Taken Within	SPEX Scores Valid for	SPEX Scores Accepted from Other Licensing Jurisdictions
Alabama	Yes	By board order	X	10 yrs	10 yrs	Yes
Alaska	Yes	To restore a retired license	X		No limit	Optional
Arizona	Yes	By board order	X	10 yrs	10 yrs	Yes
Arizona DO	Yes	By board order	X	7 yrs		
Arkansas	Yes	By board order	X			Yes
California	Yes		X	10 yrs	10 yrs	Yes
California DO	No	(COMVEX is used instead of SPEX)				
Colorado	Yes	By board order	X			Yes
Connecticut	Yes		X			Yes
Delaware	No					
DC	Yes	By board order	X			No
Florida*	Yes		X		No limit	Yes
Florida DO	No					
Georgia	Yes	By board order	X			Yes
Guam	Yes	By board order	X	10 yrs	No limit	Yes
Hawaii	Yes	If MD took a state licensing exam			No limit	Yes
Hawaii DO	No					
Idaho	Yes	By board order	X		No limit	Yes
Illinois	Yes	Restore license after disciplinary action; if not been practicing for several yrs	X		No limit	Yes
Indiana	Yes	If not been practicing; by Board order	X		No limit	Yes
Iowa	Yes	If not practicing for several yrs	X		No limit	Yes
Kansas	Yes	By board order	X		No limit	Yes
Kentucky	Yes	By board order	X		No limit	No
Louisiana	Yes		X	10 yrs	10 yrs	Yes
Maine	Yes	If not practicing for > 1 yr	X		No limit	No
Maine DO	Yes	If not practicing for > 1 yr or by board order	X		No limit	No
Maryland*	Yes	If not practicing within last 10 yrs	X	15 yrs (licensure exam) 10 yrs (ABMS exam) (or no lifetime certification)	No limit	Yes
Massachusetts	No					No
Michigan	Yes	By board order				Yes
Michigan DO	No	By board order (COMVEX is used instead of SPEX)				No
Minnesota	Yes	Restore license after disciplinary action	X	10 yrs	No limit within 3 attempts	Yes
Mississippi	Yes	Restore license after disciplinary action	X	10 yrs	10 yrs	Yes
Missouri	Yes	Restore license after disciplinary action	X		No limit	Yes
Montana	Yes	If not practicing or inactive Montana license for last 2 yrs	X	2 yrs	No limit	Yes
Nebraska	Yes		X			Yes
Nevada	Yes	To meet the 10-yr exam rule	X	10 yrs	10 yrs	Yes

Table 6 (continued)
Policies About the Special Purpose Examination

	SPEX May Be Required...	...for the Following Reasons	...to Assess Current Competence	...if Written Licensure Exam or ABMS Certification Exam Has Not Been Taken Within	SPEX Scores Valid for	SPEX Scores Accepted from Other Licensing Jurisdictions
Nevada DO	Yes	By board order	X	10 yrs	10 yrs	Yes
New Hampshire	Yes	By board order				No
New Jersey	No					No
New Mexico	Yes	Restore license after disciplinary action; if not practicing for several yrs	X		Not defined	Yes
New Mexico DO	Yes	Determined on individual basis				
New York	Yes	Determined on individual basis	X	(If state board exam taken before 1968)	No limit	Yes
North Carolina	Yes	Determined on individual basis	X	10 yrs	10 yrs	Yes
North Dakota*	Yes	(See note)	X		No limit	Yes
Ohio	Yes	If not practicing for 2 yrs	X		No limit	Yes
Oklahoma	Yes	Determined on individual basis	X			Yes
Oklahoma DO	No	(COMVEX is used instead of SPEX)	X			
Oregon	Yes	If not practicing for 1 yr, or no training or ABMS cert. for 10 yrs	X	10 yrs (or if state board exam taken before 1968)	10 yrs	Yes
Pennsylvania	Yes	Restore license after disciplinary action; if not practicing for several yrs	X			Yes
Pennsylvania DO	Yes		X			Yes
Puerto Rico	No					Yes
Rhode Island	No					No
South Carolina	Yes	Restore license after disciplinary action; if not practicing for 2 yrs	X	10 yrs	10 yrs	No
South Dakota	No					No
Tennessee	Yes	Restore license after disciplinary action; if license retired > 5 yrs	X		No limit	Yes
Tennessee DO	No					
Texas*	Yes		X	10 yrs	10 yrs	Yes
Utah	Yes	If not practicing for several yrs; restore license after discipline	X	10 yrs (DOs only)	Not defined	Yes
Vermont	No					No
Vermont DO*	Yes	Restore license if not practicing for >1 yr				
Virgin Islands	Yes	To obtain licensure	X		No limit	No
Virginia	Yes		X		No limit	No
Washington	Yes	Restore license after disciplinary action; if not practicing for 3+ yrs	X		No limit	Yes
Washington DO	Yes	If not practicing for 3 yrs	X		No limit	No
West Virginia	Yes		X		No limit	Yes
West Virginia DO	Yes		X			Yes
Wisconsin	Yes	Determined on individual basis	X		No limit	Yes
Wyoming	Yes	Determined on individual basis	X		No limit	Yes

Abbreviations

ABMS—American Board of Medical Specialties

COMVEX—Comprehensive Osteopathic Medical Variable purpose Examination

SPEX—Special Purpose Examination

* Refer to introductory text to this table for more on this state's regulations.

Note: ***All information should be verified with the licensing board; medical licenses are granted to those physicians meeting all state requirements—at the discretion of the board.***

Initial Licensure of US Medical/ Osteopathic School Graduates

All states require a written examination for initial licensure: generally, for MDs, the three-step United States Medical Licensing Examination (USMLE), which has replaced the Federation Licensing Examination (FLEX) and the national board examination of the National Board of Medical Examiners (NBME). Osteopathic physicians take the three-level Comprehensive Osteopathic Medical Licensing Examination (COMLEX-USA) of the National Board of Osteopathic Medical Examiners (NBOME).

To be eligible to take USMLE Step 3, more than half of the state medical boards require graduates of US medical schools to have completed at least 1 year of graduate medical education (GME). Twenty-three boards do not require completion of any GME to take USMLE Step 3 (although in some cases a candidate must be enrolled in a GME program).

To be eligible to take Level 3 of the Comprehensive Osteopathic Medical Licensing Examination (COMLEX), osteopathic physicians must be currently participating in and in good standing with an AOA-accredited internship or ACGME-accredited GME program or must have successfully completed such an internship or program.

All medical and osteopathic boards require completion of at least 1 year of GME before issuing a full, unrestricted license.

Table 7
Initial Licensure of US Medical/Osteopathic School Graduates

	Amount of Accredited US or Canadian GME Required	
	...to Take USMLE Step 3 or COMLEX Level 3	...for Licensure
Alabama	None (must be enrolled in GME prgm)	1 yr
Alaska	1 yr	2 yrs (1 yr if completed medical school before Jan. 1995)
Arizona	6 mos	1 yr
Arizona DO	6 mos of a 1-yr AOA- or ACGME-accredited program	1 yr AOA- or ACGME-accredited GME
Arkansas	None	1 yr
California	None	1 yr (including 4 mos general medicine)
California DO	1-yr AOA- or ACGME-accredited program	1 yr AOA- or ACGME-accredited GME, including at least 4 mos general medicine (unless applicant completed 1 yr of GME before July 1, 1990). Straight psychiatry, pathology, or anesthesiology residencies not accepted.
Colorado	1 yr	1 yr
Connecticut	None	2 yrs
Delaware	1 yr	1 yr
DC	1 yr	2 yrs
Florida	None	1 yr
Florida DO	6 mos of a 1-yr AOA- or ACGME-accredited program	1 yr AOA-approved rotating internship
Georgia	1 yr	1 yr
Guam	2 yrs	
Hawaii	None (must be enrolled in 1st year of GME prgm)	1 yr
Hawaii DO	None	1 yr AOA- or ACGME-accredited GME
Idaho	9 mos	1 yr
Illinois	1 yr	2 yrs (1 yr if entered GME before Jan. 1988)
Indiana	6 mos	1 yr
Iowa	7 mos (or enrollment in board-approved program)	1 yr AOA-, ACGME-, RCPSC-, CFPC-accredited GME
Kansas	1 yr (or enrollment in GME program in Kansas)	1 yr
Kentucky	1 yr	2 yrs
Louisiana	None	1 yr allopathic GME
Maine	1 yr	3 yrs (for those graduating after 7/1/2004)
Maine DO	1-yr AOA- or ACGME-accredited program	1 yr AOA- or ACGME-accredited GME
Maryland	None (1 yr if 3 fails on any Step)	1 yr (plus 1 yr GME if candidate failed any part of an exam 3 times)
Massachusetts	1 yr	1 yr
Michigan	6 mos	2 yrs
Michigan DO	6 mos of a 1-yr AOA- or ACGME-accredited program	1 yr AOA-approved GME
Minnesota	None (must be enrolled in GME program)	1 yr
Mississippi	1 yr	1 yr
Missouri	1 yr	1 yr
Montana	2 yrs	2 yrs
Nebraska	None	1 yr
Nevada	None	3 yrs
Nevada DO	6 mos of a 1-yr AOA- or ACGME-accredited program	3 yrs in AOA-approved or ACGME-accredited prgm (grads after 1995)

(continued on next page)

Table 7 (continued)
Initial Licensure of US Medical/Osteopathic School Graduates

	Amount of Accredited US or Canadian GME Required	
	...to Take USMLE Step 3 or COMLEX Level 3	...for Licensure
New Hampshire	1 yr	2 yrs
New Jersey	1 yr	2 yrs, and contract for year 3, if graduated after July 1, 2003; 1 yr if graduated before July 1, 2003
New Mexico	1 yr	2 yrs
New Mexico DO	6 mos of a 1-yr AOA- or ACGME-accredited program	1 yr
New York	None	1 yr
North Carolina	None	1 yr
North Dakota	6 mos of a 1-yr ACGME- or AOA-accredited program	1 yr
Ohio	9 mos	1 yr
Oklahoma	None	1 yr
Oklahoma DO	6 mos of a 1-yr AOA- or ACGME-accredited program	1 yr AOA-approved rotating internship or equivalent
Oregon	None (must be enrolled in GME program)	1 yr
Pennsylvania	None (must be enrolled in GME program)	2 yrs (1 yr if GME in US before July 1987)
Pennsylvania DO	6 mos of a 1-yr AOA- or ACGME-accredited program	1 yr AOA-approved rotating internship
Puerto Rico	None	1 yr
Rhode Island	1 yr	2 yrs
South Carolina	1 yr	1 yr
South Dakota	None	Completion of residency program
Tennessee	1 yr	1 yr
Tennessee DO	6 mos of a 1-yr AOA- or ACGME-accredited program	1-yr AOA-approved or ACGME-accredited GME
Texas	None	1 yr
Utah	None	2 yrs
Vermont	7 mos	1 yr (Canadian GME accepted if program accredited by RCPSC or CFPC)
Vermont DO	6 mos of a 1-yr AOA- or ACGME-accredited program	1 yr AOA-approved rotating internship or 3-yr AOA- or ACGME-accredited GME program
Virgin Islands	USMLE not offered	1 yr
Virginia	None	1 yr
Washington	1 yr (or enrolled in GME program)	2 yrs (1 yr if completed medical school before July 28, 1985)
Washington DO	6 mos of a 1-yr AOA- or ACGME-accredited program	1 yr AOA-approved or ACGME-accredited GME
West Virginia	None	1 yr
West Virginia DO	1-yr AOA- or ACGME-accredited program	1 yr AOA-approved GME
Wisconsin	1 yr	1 yr
Wyoming	1 yr	1 yr

Abbreviations

USMLE—United States Medical Licensing Examination

COMLEX—Comprehensive Osteopathic Medical Licensing Examination

GME—graduate medical education

RCPSC—Royal College of Physicians and Surgeons of Canada

Note: ***All information should be verified with the licensing board; medical licenses are granted to those physicians meeting all state requirements—at the discretion of the board.***

Initial Licensure of Canadian Citizens Who Are Graduates of Accredited Canadian Medical Schools

When considering applications for licensure, all state medical boards consider Canadian citizens who have graduated from an accredited Canadian medical school on the same basis as graduates of accredited US medical schools.

Forty-seven licensing boards endorse the Licentiate of the Medical Council of Canada (LMCC) as evidence of passing an acceptable licensing examination (applicants must also pass all other board requirements for licensure).

With the exception of Guam and the Virgin Islands, all licensing boards accept Canadian graduate medical education (GME) as equivalent to GME in a US program accredited by the Accreditation Council for Graduate Medical Education (ACGME). These rules do not uniformly apply to international medical graduates, who should refer to Table 9.

Table 8
Initial Licensure of Canadian Citizens Who Are Graduates of Accredited Canadian Medical Schools

	LMCC Approved for Licensure by Endorsement	GME in Accredited Canadian Programs Accepted as Equivalent to ACGME-accredited GME in the United States	Notes
Alabama	Yes	Yes	
Alaska	Yes	Yes	
Arizona	Yes	Yes	
Arkansas	Yes	Yes	
California	Yes	Yes	
Colorado	Yes	Yes	
Connecticut	Yes	Yes	
Delaware	Yes	Yes	
DC	Yes	Yes	
Florida	No	Yes	
Georgia	Yes	Yes	
Guam	No	No	
Hawaii	No	Yes	
Idaho	Yes	Yes	
Illinois	Yes	Yes	
Indiana	Yes	Yes	
Iowa	Yes	Yes	LMCC must be endorsed by provincial licensing board
Kansas	Yes	Yes	
Kentucky	Yes	Yes	
Louisiana	No	Yes	
Maine	Yes	Yes	
Maryland	Yes	Yes	
Massachusetts	Yes	Yes	
Michigan	Yes	Yes	
Minnesota	Yes	Yes	
Mississippi	Yes	Yes	
Missouri	Yes	Yes	Only if medical school graduate of Canadian medical school
Montana	Yes	Yes	
Nebraska	Yes	Yes	
Nevada	Yes	Yes	
New Hampshire	Yes	Yes	
New Jersey	No	Yes	LMCC considered *only* if applicant is licensed in US jurisdiction
New Mexico	Yes	Yes	
New York	Yes	Yes	LMCC considered *only* if applicant has valid provincial license
North Carolina	Yes	Yes	
North Dakota	Yes	Yes	
Ohio	Yes	Yes	1 yr of GME or its equivalent required

Table 8 (continued)
Initial Licensure of Canadian Citizens Who Are Graduates of Accredited Canadian Medical Schools

	LMCC Approved for Licensure by Endorsement	GME in Accredited Canadian Programs Accepted as Equivalent to ACGME-accredited GME in the United States	Notes
Oklahoma	Yes	Yes	
Oregon	Yes	Yes	
Pennsylvania	Yes	Yes	Must have received LMCC after 5/70 and in English
Puerto Rico	No	Yes	LMCC considered *only* if applicant is licensed in US jurisdiction
Rhode Island	Yes	Yes	
South Carolina	Yes	Yes	
South Dakota	Yes	Yes	
Tennessee	Yes	Yes	
Texas	Yes	Yes	
Utah	Yes	Yes	
Vermont	Yes	Yes	
Virgin Islands	No	No	
Virginia	Yes	Yes	
Washington	Yes	Yes	Must have received LMCC after 12/69
West Virginia	Yes	Yes	
Wisconsin	Yes	Yes	Must have received LMCC after 1/1/78
Wyoming	Yes	Yes	

Abbreviations

ACGME—Accreditation Council for Graduate Medical Education

GME—graduate medical education

LMCC—certification by the Licentiate of the Medical Council of Canada

Note: ***All information should be verified with the licensing board; licenses based on endorsement are granted to those physicians meeting all state requirements.***

Initial Licensure of International Medical Graduates

All international medical graduates (IMGs) must hold a certificate from the Educational Commission for Foreign Medical Graduates (ECFMG) examination before taking Step 3 of the United States Medical Licensing Examination (USMLE). (For more information on the ECFMG certificate, see p. 98.)

Eighteen boards maintain and use a list of approved/unapproved foreign medical schools for initial licensure decisions. New Mexico and Tennessee use the list of schools from the California board. In addition, about half of the boards require IMG candidates for endorsement of licensure to have graduated from a state-approved foreign medical school (see Table 5, column 3).

Thirty-nine states will endorse for licensure the Licentiate of the Medical Council of Canada (LMCC) when held by an IMG.

Eighteen state boards allow IMGs to take USMLE Step 3 before they have had GME in a US or Canadian hospital. All states, however, require at least 1 year of GME for licensure, and 30 states require 3 years. Candidates are not awarded a license until they undertake the required GME in the United States and meet other board requirements (eg, an ECFMG certificate, personal interview, payment of fees).

Fifth Pathway

In 1971, the AMA established Fifth Pathway, a program for US citizens studying abroad at foreign medical schools. The program requires that participants have

1. Completed, in an accredited US college or university, undergraduate premedical work of a quality acceptable for matriculation in an accredited US medical school, evaluated by measures such as college grade point average and scores on the Medical College Admission Test
2. Studied medicine in a foreign medical school located outside the US, including Puerto Rico, and Canada that is listed in the *International Medical Education Directory*, available on the ECFMG Web site at www.ecfmg.org and developed and maintained by the Foundation for Advancement of International Medical Education and Research (FAIMER^{SM}), a nonprofit foundation of the ECFMG
3. Completed all formal requirements for a diploma of the foreign medical school except internship and/or social service (Those who have completed all the formal graduation requirements of the foreign medical school, including internship and/or social service, and are consequently eligible to apply for ECFMG certification, are not eligible for the Fifth Pathway.)

If the aforementioned criteria are met, the candidate may substitute the Fifth Pathway program for internship and/or social service in the foreign country. After receiving a Fifth Pathway certificate from an accredited US medical school, these US citizens are eligible to enter the first year of GME in the United States.

In 52 jurisdictions (exceptions are Guam and the Virgin Islands), individuals who hold Fifth Pathway certificates (but not the ECFMG certificate) are eligible for licensure. Fifth Pathway certificate holders must pass Steps 1 and 2 of the USMLE before entering a GME program accredited by the Accreditation Council for Graduate Medical Education (ACGME).

Additional Notes for Specific Licensing Jurisdictions

Florida—ECFMG certificate required for licensure if a candidate is not a graduate of a foreign medical school approved by the Florida Board of Medicine (none has yet been approved).

Maine—GME taken in Canada or the British Isles (accredited by a national body deemed equivalent to ACGME) may be considered qualifying on an individual basis.

Maryland—In addition to 2 years of ACGME- or AOA-accredited GME required for licensure, 1 year of GME required if a candidate failed any part of an examination three times; no more than three failures permitted.

Mississippi—ABMS board certification required for candidates who completed the Fifth Pathway.

New Jersey—An individual's educational experience must meet certain eligibility requirements.

North Carolina—Less than 3 years of GME may be accepted if applicant has completed at least 1 year of approved GME and is certified by an ABMS or AOA specialty board.

North Dakota—Three years of US or Canadian GME is required for licensure; if a candidate has not completed 3 years of GME but has met all other licensing requirements and has completed 1 year of GME in the United States or Canada in a board-approved program, and if the board finds that the candidate has other professional experience and training substantially equivalent to the second and third years of GME, the candidate may be deemed eligible for licensure (upon passing SPEX or ABMS board certification).

Oregon—IMG candidates for licensure must have completed at least 3 years of progressive GME in not more than two specialties in not more than two US or Canadian hospitals accredited for such training.

Pennsylvania—The board will grant unrestricted license by endorsement to a candidate who does not meet standard requirements if the candidate has achieved cumulative qualifications that are endorsed by the board as being equivalent to the standard license requirements.

South Carolina—ABMS/AOA board certification required for candidates who completed the Fifth Pathway.

South Dakota—No list of approved/unapproved foreign medical schools is maintained; decisions made on a case-by-case basis.

Table 9
Initial Licensure of International Medical Graduates

	Accepts Fifth Pathway	Maintains/ Uses List of Approved Foreign Med Schools	Endorses Canadian Certificate (LMCC) Held by an IMG	Amount of Accredited US or Canadian GME Required	
				...to Take USMLE Step 3	...for Licensure
Alabama	Yes	Yes	Yes	2 yrs (must be in 3rd yr of GME)	3 yrs
Alaska	Yes	Yes	Yes	1 yr	3 yrs
Arizona	Yes	No	Yes	6 mos	3 yrs
Arkansas	Yes	Yes	Yes	None	3 yrs (1 yr if currently enrolled in prgm at U of Arkansas for Med Sci)
California	Yes		Yes	None	2 yrs (including 4 mos general med)
Colorado	Yes	Yes	Yes/No (case-by-case review)	3 yrs	3 yrs
Connecticut	Yes	Yes (WHO)	Yes	None	2 yrs
Delaware	Yes	No	No	1 yr	3 yrs
DC	Yes	No	Yes	3 yrs	3 yrs
Florida*	Yes	No	No	None	2 yrs
Georgia	Yes	No	Yes	1-3 yrs	3 yrs
Guam	No	No	No	2 yrs	3 yrs
Hawaii	Yes	No	No	1 yr (must be in 2nd yr of pgm)	2 yrs
Idaho	Yes	Yes	No	2 yrs, 9 mos	3 yrs
Illinois	Yes	No	Yes	1 yr	1 yr (entered GME pre-1988); 2 yrs (entered GME post-1988)
Indiana	Yes	Yes	Yes	2 yrs	2 yrs
Iowa	Yes	No	Yes (with valid Canadian provincial license and fulfillment of all other licensure requirements)	7 mos (or enrollment in GME pgm approved by board at time of application for Step 3)	2 yrs AOA-, ACGME-, RCPSC-, or CFPC-accredited GME
Kansas	Yes	Yes	Yes	2 yrs (or enrollment in GME program in Kansas)	2 yrs
Kentucky	Yes	No	Yes	1 yr	2 yrs
Louisiana	Yes	Yes (WHO)	No	None	3 yrs (Fifth Pathway may be counted as 1 yr of required GME)
Maine*	Yes	Yes (IMED)	Yes	2 yrs	3 yrs
Maryland*	Yes	No	Yes	None (1 yr if 3 fails on any Step)	2 yrs AOA- or ACGME-accredited GME (as of Oct. 1, 2000)
Massachusetts	Yes	No	Yes	1 yr	2 yrs
Michigan	Yes	No	Yes (with valid Canadian license)	6 mos	2 yrs
Minnesota	Yes	Yes	Yes	None (must be in GME program)	2 yrs
Mississippi*	Yes	No	No	3 yrs	3 yrs (or 1 yr plus ABMS certification)
Missouri	Yes	No	No	3 yrs	3 yrs
Montana	Yes	Yes	No	3 yrs	3 yrs (or ABMS or AOA certification)
Nebraska	Yes	No	Yes	None	3 yrs
Nevada	Yes	No	Yes	None	3 yrs
New Hampshire	Yes	No	Yes	1 yr	2 yrs
New Jersey*	Yes	Yes (WHO)*	No	1 yr	3 yrs (1 yr if medical school completed before July 1, 1985); 2 yrs, and contract for year 3, if graduated after July 1, 2003

Table 9 (continued)
Initial Licensure of International Medical Graduates

	Accepts Fifth Pathway	Maintains/ Uses List of Approved Foreign Med Schools	Endorses Canadian Certificate (LMCC) Held by an IMG	Amount of Accredited US or Canadian GME Required	
				...to Take USMLE Step 3	...for Licensure
New Mexico	Yes	Yes (CA list)	No	1 yr	2 yrs
New York	Yes	No	Yes (with valid Canadian provincial license and fulfillment of all other licensure requirements)	None	3 yrs
North Carolina	Yes	No	Yes	3 yrs (none if enrolled in-state)	3 yrs
North Dakota*	Yes	Yes	Yes	1 yr (none if enrolled in-state)	3 yrs
Ohio	Yes	No	Yes	9 mos	2 yrs (through the 2nd-yr level)
Oklahoma	Yes	No	Yes	None	2 yrs
Oregon*	Yes	No	Yes	None (must be in GME program)	3 yrs
Pennsylvania*	Yes	No	Yes (if passed after 5/70 and in English)	None (must be in GME program)	3 yrs (1 yr if GME taken in US before July 1987)
Puerto Rico	Yes		Yes	None	1 yr
Rhode Island	Yes	Yes (WHO)	Yes (with valid Canadian provincial license and fulfillment of all other licensure requirements)	1 yr	3 yrs
South Carolina*	Yes	No	Yes	3 yrs	3 yrs
South Dakota*	Yes	No	Yes	1 yr	Completion of residency (1 yr if US GME taken before 7/87)
Tennessee	Yes	Yes (CA list)	Yes	1 yr	3 yrs
Texas	Yes	Yes	Yes	None	3 yrs
Utah	Yes	No	No	None	2 yrs
Vermont	Yes	Yes	No	7 mos	3 yrs (Canadian GME not accepted)
Virgin Islands	No	No	No	Not applicable	1 yr US GME
Virginia	Yes	No	Yes	None	2 yrs
Washington	Yes	No	Yes (if passed after 12/69)	1 yr (or enrollment in GME program)	2 yrs (1 yr if medical school completed before July 28, 1985)
West Virginia	Yes	No	Yes	None	3 yrs (or 1 yr plus ABMS cert.)
Wisconsin	Yes	No	Yes (if passed after 12/77)	1 yr	1 yr
Wyoming*	Yes	No	Yes	2 yrs	2 yrs

Abbreviations

GME—graduate medical education

IMED—*International Medical Education Directory*

IMG—international medical graduate

LMCC—Licentiate of the Medical Council of Canada

USMLE—United States Medical Licensing Examination

WHO—World Health Organization

* Refer to introductory text to this table for more information on this state's regulations.

Note: ***All information should be verified with the licensing board; licenses are granted to those physicians meeting all state requirements—at the discretion of the board.***

Medical Student Clerkship Regulations

For purposes of this publication, a clerkship is defined as clinical education provided to medical students. Twenty states evaluate the quality of clinical clerkships in connection with an application for licensure. In most states, clerkships for US medical students must take place in hospitals affiliated with medical schools accredited by the Liaison Committee on Medical Education (LCME). Eleven states have additional and/or more specific bases for evaluation.

Twelve boards regulate clerkships provided in their states to students of foreign medical schools (including US citizens studying medicine in foreign schools). Of these, Pennsylvania and Puerto Rico forbid such clerkships. For purposes of licensure, 20 states accept only those clerkships completed in hospital departments with graduate medical education (GME) programs accredited by the Accreditation Council for Graduate Medical Education (ACGME). Eight states have additional regulations.

Additional Notes for Specific Licensing Jurisdictions

California—Students of foreign medical schools may complete up to 18 of 72 required weeks in nonapproved clerkships outside of California.

Florida—Rules on clinical clerkships for international medical graduates adopted by the Florida Board before October 1986 do not apply to any graduate who had already completed a clinical clerkship or who had begun a clinical clerkship, as long as the clerkship was completed within 3 years.

An international medical school must be registered with the Florida Department of Education for its students to perform clinical clerkships in Florida.

Michigan—Specific clerkships are required (only for MDs, not DOs).

Texas—Clerkships must be performed 1) as a student in an accredited medical or osteopathic school or 2) in a hospital or teaching institution sponsoring or participating in a GME program accredited by the ACGME, the AOA, or the board in the same specialty or subspecialty as the medical or osteopathic medical education. The only exception is for applicants who are ABMS or AOA Bureau of Osteopathic Specialists specialty board certified.

Table 10
Medical Student Clerkship Regulations

	Evaluates the Quality of Clinical Clerkships in Connection with a Licensure Application	Regulation of Clerkships Provided to Students of Foreign Medical Schools			
		Regulates Clerkships Provided by Hospitals	Forbids Clerkships for Students of Foreign Med. Schools	Accepts Clerkships Only in Hospital Departments with ACGME-accredited Programs	Has Additional Regulations
Alabama	Yes			Yes	
Alaska					
Arizona					
Arkansas	Yes†	Yes		Yes	
California*	Yes†	Yes		Yes	Yes
Colorado					
Connecticut	Yes†	Yes		Yes	
Delaware	Yes	Yes		Yes	
DC				Yes	
Florida*	Yes	Yes		Yes	Yes
Georgia	Yes†			Yes	
Guam	Yes			Yes	
Hawaii					
Idaho					
Illinois					
Indiana					
Iowa					
Kansas					
Kentucky	Yes			Yes	
Louisiana					
Maine				Yes	
Maryland					
Massachusetts	Yes†	Yes		Yes	Yes
Michigan*					Yes
Minnesota					
Mississippi					
Missouri					
Montana					
Nebraska					
Nevada					
New Hampshire					
New Jersey	Yes†	Yes		Yes	Yes
New Mexico	Yes†				
New York	Yes†	Yes		Yes	Yes
North Carolina					
North Dakota					
Ohio					
Oklahoma				Yes	
Oregon	Yes	Yes		Yes	
Pennsylvania	Yes†	Yes	Yes	Yes	

(continued on next page)

Table 10 (continued)
Medical Student Clerkship Regulations

	Evaluates the Quality of Clinical Clerkships in Connection with a Licensure Application	Regulation of Clerkships Provided to Students of Foreign Medical Schools			
		Regulates Clerkships Provided by Hospitals	Forbids Clerkships for Students of Foreign Med. Schools	Accepts Clerkships Only in Hospital Departments with ACGME-accredited Programs	Has Additional Regulations
Puerto Rico	Yes	Yes	Yes		
Rhode Island	Yes			Yes	
South Carolina					
South Dakota					
Tennessee					
Texas*	Yes†	Yes		Yes	Yes
Utah					
Vermont					
Virgin Islands					
Virginia	Yes†			Yes	
Washington					
West Virginia					
Wisconsin					
Wyoming	Yes				Yes
Total	**20**	**12**	**2**	**20**	**8**

* Refer to introductory text to this table for more information on this state's regulations.

† In many cases, clerkships must take place in hospitals affiliated with LCME-accredited medical schools or ACGME-accredited residency programs. These states require additional and/or more specific criteria for evaluation.

Note: ***All information should be verified with the licensing board; medical licenses are granted to those physicians meeting all state requirements—at the discretion of the board.***

Additional Policies Concerning IMGs and DOs

A number of state medical boards have additional graduate medical education (GME) and specialty certificate policies for international medical graduates (IMGs). Fifteen states have requirements for appointment to GME programs other than requiring an Educational Commission for Foreign Medical Graduates (ECFMG) certificate or a limited license.

Six boards—Connecticut, Maine, Nebraska, Ohio, Oklahoma, and Rhode Island—indicated that GME completed in foreign countries other than Canada may be considered for credit toward a license. Specialty certificates of foreign boards, such as the Royal College of Physicians in the United Kingdom, may be accepted for credit toward a license in 11 states.

Thirty-six medical boards accept GME accredited by the Accreditation Council for Graduate Medical Education (ACGME) for licensure of osteopathic medical graduates.

Additional Notes for Specific Licensing Jurisdictions

Maine—The board may accept GME completed in England, Scotland, and Ireland for credit toward a license, if it is accepted by the specialty board as meeting board eligibility in the United States and notified via certified letter.

Pennsylvania—IMGs seeking appointment to a GME program need a passing score on United States Medical Licensing Examination (USMLE) Steps 1 and 2 (or National Board of Medical Examiners [NBME] Parts I and II or Federation Licensing Examination [FLEX] Component 1) for graduate year 2 medical education; for graduate year 3 and beyond, all parts of USMLE (or NBME or FLEX) are required.

Table 11
Additional Policies Concerning IMGs and DOs

	Has State Board Requirements for Appointment to GME Program Other Than ECFMG Certificate or Limited License	May Accept GME Completed in Foreign Countries Other Than Canada for Credit Toward a License	May Accept Specialty Certificates of Foreign Boards (eg, Royal College of Physicians of the United Kingdom) for Credit Toward a License	Osteopathic Medical Graduates	
				ACGME-Accredited GME Accepted	State Osteopathic Board Handles Licensure
Alabama				Yes	
Alaska	Yes (residency permit required)				
Arizona	Yes (residency permit required)				Yes
Arkansas				Yes	
California	Yes				Yes
Colorado				Yes	
Connecticut	Yes (residency intern permit required)	Yes	Yes	Yes	
Delaware					
DC				Yes	
Florida					Yes
Georgia				Yes	
Guam					
Hawaii					
Idaho				Yes	
Illinois				Yes	
Indiana				Yes	
Iowa				Yes	
Kansas	Yes (residency permit required, and unapproved school must have been in existence at least 15 yrs)			Yes	
Kentucky	Yes (residency permit required for 2nd yr)			Yes	
Louisiana	Yes (passage of FLEX/NBME/USMLE)			Yes	
Maine*		Yes	Yes	Yes	Yes
Maryland				Yes	
Massachusetts				Yes	
Michigan	Yes (certification of medical education)				Yes
Minnesota	Yes (residency intern permit required)			Yes	
Mississippi				Yes	
Missouri	Yes			Yes	
Montana				Yes	
Nebraska		Yes		Yes	
Nevada	Yes				Yes
New Hampshire				Yes	
New Jersey	Yes (residency intern permit required)			Yes	
New Mexico					Yes
New York			Yes	Yes	
North Carolina				Yes	
North Dakota				Yes	
Ohio		Yes	Yes	Yes	

Table 11 (continued)
Additional Policies Concerning IMGs and DOs

	Has State Board Requirements for Appointment to GME Program Other Than ECFMG Certificate or Limited License	May Accept GME Completed in Foreign Countries Other Than Canada for Credit Toward a License	May Accept Specialty Certificates of Foreign Boards (eg, Royal College of Physicians of the United Kingdom) for Credit Toward a License	Osteopathic Medical Graduates	
				ACGME-Accredited GME Accepted	State Osteopathic Board Handles Licensure
Oklahoma		Yes	Yes		Yes
Oregon				Yes	
Pennsylvania*	Yes		Yes		Yes
Puerto Rico					
Rhode Island		Yes (UK only)	Yes; may accept certificates of boards in England, Scotland, and Ireland	Yes	
South Carolina				Yes	
South Dakota				Yes	
Tennessee			Yes; specialty board must be AMA-recognized		Yes
Texas	Yes (physician-in-training permit required)			Yes	
Utah				Yes	Yes
Vermont	Yes		Yes; specialty board must be recognized by ABMS, RCPSC, or CFPC		Yes
Virgin Islands					
Virginia					
Washington				Yes	Yes
West Virginia				Yes	
Wisconsin			Yes		
Wyoming			Yes (at board's discretion)	Yes	
Total	**15**	**6**	**11**	**36**	**13**

Abbreviations

ACGME—Accreditation Council for Graduate Medical Education
ECFMG—Educational Commission for Foreign Medical Graduates
FLEX—Federation Licensing Examination
GME—graduate medical education
NBME—certificate of the National Board of Medical Examiners
USMLE—United States Medical Licensing Examination

* Refer to introductory text to this table for more information on this state's regulations.

Note: ***All information should be verified with the licensing board; medical licenses are granted to those physicians meeting all state requirements—at the discretion of the board.***

Accredited Subspecialties and Nonaccredited Fellowships That Satisfy GME Requirements for Licensure

Both the AMA and the Accreditation Council for Graduate Medical Education (ACGME) define a residency as graduate medical education (GME) that takes place in any of the medical specialties with ACGME Program Requirements (eg, internal medicine, pediatrics, surgery). Beginning in 2000, the ACGME has used the term *fellowship* to denote GME in ACGME-accredited subspecialty programs (eg, cardiovascular disease, vascular surgery, rheumatology) that is beyond the requirements for eligibility for first board certification in the discipline.

All state medical boards accept residency education in specialty programs accredited by the ACGME as satisfying their GME requirements for licensure. Fifty-one jurisdictions—all except Arkansas, Montana, and Puerto Rico—accept residency education in subspecialty programs accredited by ACGME as satisfying their GME requirements for licensure.

Eight boards accept clinical fellowships not accredited by ACGME, and three boards—Hawaii, New York, and North Carolina—may accept (with board approval, in some cases) research fellowships not accredited by ACGME to satisfy the GME requirement for licensure.

Table 12
Accredited Subspecialties and Nonaccredited Fellowships That Satisfy Graduate Medical Education Requirements for Licensure

	Accepts Subspecialty GME Accredited by ACGME	Accepts Clinical Fellowships ***Not*** Accredited by ACGME	Accepts Research Fellowships ***Not*** Accredited by ACGME
Alabama	Yes (if clinical)		
Alaska	Yes		
Arizona	Yes		
Arkansas			
California MD and DO	Yes		
Colorado	Yes		
Connecticut	Yes		
Delaware	Yes		
DC	Yes		
Florida	Yes		
Georgia	Yes	Yes	
Guam	Yes		
Hawaii	Yes	Yes	Yes
Idaho	Yes		
Illinois	Yes		
Indiana	Yes		
Iowa	Yes		
Kansas	Yes		
Kentucky	Yes		
Louisiana	Yes		
Maine	Yes		
Maryland	Yes		
Massachusetts	Yes		
Michigan	Yes		
Michigan DO	Only if AOA-accredited		
Minnesota	Yes		
Mississippi	Yes		
Missouri	Yes	Yes	
Montana			
Nebraska	Yes		
Nevada	Yes		
New Hampshire	Yes		
New Jersey	Yes		
New Mexico	Yes		
New York	Yes	Yes	Yes
North Carolina	Yes	Yes (with board approval)	Yes (with board approval)
North Dakota	Yes		
Ohio	Yes	Yes (with board approval)	
Oklahoma	Yes		
Oregon	Yes		
Pennsylvania	Yes		
Puerto Rico			
Rhode Island	Yes	Yes (with board approval)	
South Carolina	Yes		
South Dakota	Yes		

(continued on next page)

Table 12 (continued)
Accredited Subspecialties and Nonaccredited Fellowships That Satisfy Graduate Medical Education Requirements for Licensure

	Accepts Subspecialty GME Accredited by ACGME	Accepts Clinical Fellowships ***Not*** Accredited by ACGME	Accepts Research Fellowships ***Not*** Accredited by ACGME
Tennessee	Yes		
Texas	Yes	Yes (if in Texas and board-approved)	
Utah	Yes	Yes (if combined with an ACGME-accredited program)	
Vermont	Yes		
Virgin Islands	Yes		
Virginia	Yes		
Washington MD and DO	Yes		
West Virginia	Yes		
Wisconsin	Yes		
Wyoming	Yes		
Total	**51**	**9**	**3**

Abbreviations

ACGME—Accreditation Council for Graduate Medical Education
GME—graduate medical education

* Refer to introductory text to this table for more information on this state's regulations.

Note: ***All information should be verified with licensing board; medical licenses are granted to those physicians meeting all state requirements—at the discretion of the board.***

Licensure Requirement Exemptions for Eminent Physicians and Medical School Faculty

Fifteen boards license physicians through recognition of eminence in medical education or medical practice. Physicians appointed to a medical school faculty are excused from the graduate medical education (GME) requirement for limited licensure in 18 states and from the examination requirement for limited licensure or teaching certification in 17 states. These faculty appointees would, however, receive a limited license or similar credential.

Table 13
Licensure Requirement Exemptions for Eminent Physicians and Medical School Faculty

	License Physicians Through Recognition of Eminence in Medical Education or Practice	Physicians Appointed to a Medical Faculty Are Excused From...		Notes/Comments
		...the GME Requirement for Limited Licensure	...the Examination Requirement for Limited Licensure	
Alabama		Yes	Yes	
Alaska				
Arizona				
Arkansas				
California DO	Yes	Yes	Yes	
California MD	Yes	Yes	Yes	1-yr medical faculty certificate, for practice only at the medical school or a formally affiliated teaching hospital
Colorado				Distinguished foreign physicians are invited to serve on faculty; temporary licensure may not exceed 5 years
Connecticut		Yes	Yes	
Delaware				
DC	Yes			
Florida		Yes	Yes	Physicians appointed to a medical faculty are eligible for a special license, with which they may practice only at the designated facility/institution
Georgia		Yes	Yes	Physicians appointed to a medical faculty are excused from the GME requirement for limited licensure for teaching only
Guam				
Hawaii				
Idaho				
Illinois				
Indiana				
Iowa	Yes	Yes	Yes	Physicians appointed to a medical faculty are eligible for a special license, with which they may practice only at the designated facility/institution. Time spent on a special license can be applied to the GME requirements for permanent licensure
Kansas				
Kentucky	Yes	Yes	Yes	Physicians appointed to a medical faculty are eligible for a special license, with which they may practice only at the designated facility/institution
Louisiana	Yes	Yes	Yes	A physician licensed through recognition of eminence in medical education must be approved as a tenured professor/associate professor by a Louisiana medical school
Maine				
Maryland	Yes	Yes	Yes	
Massachusetts				
Michigan				
Minnesota				
Mississippi				
Missouri	Yes		Yes	
Montana	Yes			An IMG seeking a restricted license must have published in an English-language, peer-reviewed medical journal
Nebraska				
Nevada				
New Hampshire	Yes			A courtesy license for educational purposes is provided to eminent physicians under limited circumstances

(continued on next page)

Table 13 (continued)
Licensure Requirement Exemptions for Eminent Physicians and Medical School Faculty

	License Physicians Through Recognition of Eminence in Medical Education or Practice	Physicians Appointed to a Medical Faculty Are Excused From…		Notes/Comments
		…the GME Requirement for Limited Licensure	…the Examination Requirement for Limited Licensure	
New Jersey				
New Mexico				
New York				
North Carolina	Yes	Yes	Yes	Also excused from ECFMG certification requirement
North Dakota				
Ohio		Yes	Yes	Physicians appointed to a medical faculty are eligible for a visiting medical faculty certificate, with which they may practice only at the school or teaching hospitals affiliated with the school. This nonrenewable certificate is valid 1 year or duration of the appointment, whichever is shorter
Oklahoma				
Oregon		Yes		IMGs who are not eligible for licensure may be granted a Limited License, Medical Faculty (LL,MF) if appointed to a full-time medical school faculty position under direction of the department head. LL,MF may be granted annually for 4 years, during which the applicant must pass USMLE Steps 1, 2, and 3 or have passed FLEX or the National Boards. The physician would then be eligible for licensure.
Pennsylvania DO				
Pennsylvania MD	Yes	Yes		Physicians appointed to a medical faculty are eligible for a visiting medical faculty certificate, with which they may practice only at the school or teaching hospitals affiliated with the school. This nonrenewable certificate is valid 1 year or duration of the appointment, whichever is shorter
Puerto Rico				
Rhode Island	Yes	Yes	Yes	Distinguished foreign physicians recommended by the medical school dean may serve on faculty; academic limited registration may be renewed for a maximum of 5 years
South Carolina				
South Dakota				
Tennessee		Yes	Yes	
Texas	Yes	See note	See note	There are several types of limited licenses, each with differ ent requirements and characteristics. Contact the board for more information.
Utah				
Vermont		Yes	Yes	
Virgin Islands				
Virginia				
Washington				
West Virginia		Yes	Yes	
Wisconsin				
Wyoming	Yes			Exemption granted at Board's discretion
Total	**15**	**18**	**17**	

Note: ***All information should be verified with licensing board; medical licenses are granted to those physicians meeting all state requirements—at the discretion of the board.***

Teaching (Visiting Professor) Licenses

Thirty-nine jurisdictions issue teaching (visiting professor) licenses, with fees ranging from $0 to $400.

Table 14
Teaching (Visiting Professor) Licenses

	Teaching (Visiting Professor) License Granted	Notes
Alabama	Yes	
Alaska		
Arizona	Yes, $100	Teaching licenses, for practice within clinical training program only, granted to full-time faculty members at accredited med school or GME program ($225)
Arizona DO	Yes, $318	Education Training Permit, granted for 5 days, $106
Arkansas	Yes, $400	Education license must be renewed annually
California	Yes	Renewable certificates of registration are awarded on an individual basis for 1 to 5 years to physicians who do not immediately meet licensure requirements and who have been offered full-time teaching positions in California medical schools. Biennially renewable faculty permits are awarded on an individual basis to academically eminent physicians for whom the medical school has assumed direct responsibility. The holder may practice medicine only within the sponsoring medical school and affiliated institutions.
California DO		
Colorado	Yes, $100	
Connecticut	Yes, $0	
Delaware		
DC		
Florida	Yes, $100	A visiting faculty certificate, valid for 180 days, is granted to MDs/DOs who are graduates of an accredited medical school or its equivalent and hold a valid current license to practice medicine in another US jurisdiction. The certificate authorizes practice only in conjunction with teaching duties at an accredited Florida medical/osteopathic school or in its main teaching hospitals. No more than three physicians per year per institution may hold this certificate; the certificate can be granted to a physician only once in a given 5-year period.
Florida DO	Yes, $400	(See above note)
Georgia	Yes	Teacher's license for faculty of approved Georgia medical schools.
Guam		
Hawaii		
Hawaii DO		
Idaho		
Illinois	Yes	Visiting Professor Permits for a maximum of 2 years are issued to persons receiving faculty appointments to teach in either a medical or osteopathic school. Visiting Physician Permits for up to 180 days are issued to persons receiving an invitation or appointment to study, demonstrate, or perform a specific medical or osteopathic subject or technique in medical/osteopathic schools; hospitals; or facilities operated pursuant to the Ambulatory Surgical Treatment Center Act.
Indiana	Yes, $100	Visiting professor license granted to an institution for a specific physician to whom it has granted a visiting faculty appointment. Institution must certify the physician's qualifications; physician's practice limited to the institution for designated period not to exceed 1 yr
Iowa	Yes, $346	
Kansas	Yes, $25	
Kentucky	Yes, $250	
Louisiana	Yes	
Maine	Yes, $0	
Maine DO		
Maryland	Yes, $334	Limited 1-yr license for graduate teaching
Massachusetts	Yes, $250	Temporary registration is issued to physicians who hold a temporary faculty appointment at a Massachusetts medical school, are substituting temporarily for a fully licensed Massachusetts physician, or are enrolled in a CME course that requires Massachusetts licensure. Physicians requesting temporary registration must be currently licensed in another state.

Table 14 (continued)
Teaching (Visiting Professor) Licenses

	Teaching (Visiting Professor) License Granted	Notes
Michigan	Yes, $170	
Michigan DO	Yes	
Minnesota		
Mississippi		
Missouri	Yes	
Montana		Refer to 37-3-305, MCA
Nebraska	Yes, $25	Temporary visiting faculty permits for medical school faculty
Nevada		
Nevada DO	Yes, $200	
New Hampshire	Yes, $75	
New Jersey		
New Mexico	Yes, $100	
New Mexico DO		
New York		
North Carolina	Yes, $150	Limited faculty license for medical school faculty
North Dakota		
Ohio	Yes, $125	Visiting Medical Faculty certificate and Special Activities certificates are $125
Oklahoma		
Oklahoma DO		
Oregon	Yes, $175	Limited license (LL) is issued for Visiting Professor (VP) and Medical Faculty (MF). LL-VP is valid for a 1-year teaching position and may be renewed for 1 additional year. LL-MF is valid for a full-time faculty position offered by the dean of the medical school and may be renewed for 3 additional years.
Pennsylvania	Yes	Institutional License allows a qualified person to teach and/or practice medicine for a period of time not to exceed 3 years in one of the Commonwealth's medical colleges, its affiliates, or community hospitals. Temporary License allows the licensee to teach medicine and surgery or participate in a medical procedure necessary for the well-being of a specified patient within the Commonwealth. Applicants for a temporary license must hold an unrestricted license in another state, territory, possession, or country.
Pennsylvania DO		
Puerto Rico	Yes	
Rhode Island	Yes, $150	
South Carolina		
South Dakota		Teaching or visiting professor licenses, permits, or certificates are not issued
Tennessee	Yes, $50	
Tennessee DO		
Texas	Yes, $110	
Utah		
Vermont		
Vermont DO		
Virgin Islands	Yes	
Virginia	Yes, $55	Limited license for fellowship and teaching positions

Table 14 (continued)
Teaching (Visiting Professor) Licenses

	Teaching (Visiting Professor) License Granted	Notes
Washington	Yes	Teaching (visiting professor) license for teaching/research at state institutions or city/county health fellowships, only to physicians currently licensed in another state or country
Washington DO		
West Virginia	Yes, $150	
West Virginia DO		
Wisconsin	Yes, $110	
Wyoming		
Total	**39**	

Note: ***All information should be verified with licensing board; medical licenses are granted to those physicians meeting all state requirements—at the discretion of the board.***

Licensure and Reregistration Fees and Intervals; CME Reporting Requirements

The National Board of Medical Examiners (NBME) administers United States Medical Licensing Examination (USMLE) Steps 1 and 2 to students and graduates of US and Canadian medical schools at test centers established by the NBME; application materials are usually available at these medical schools. The Educational Commission for Foreign Medical Graduates (ECFMG) administers USMLE Steps 1 and 2 to students and graduates of foreign medical schools; application materials are available only through the ECFMG.

Administration of USMLE Step 3 is the responsibility of the individual medical licensing jurisdictions. Step 3 application materials for physicians who have successfully completed Steps 1 and 2 are available from the medical licensing authorities or the Federation of State Medical Boards (FSMB), which administers the examination for all jurisdictions, except Florida, Guam, and the Virgin Islands. (For more information on USMLE Step 3, call 800 USMLE XM—800 876-5396). Although the FSMB administers the examination, in six jurisdictions (Alabama, District of Columbia, Illinois, Missouri, Puerto Rico, and Wisconsin) physicians apply for the examination directly via the state board rather than by way of the FSMB.

The fee for 2007 for USMLE Step 3 is $655; exceptions for 2006 (2007 exceptions are not yet available) are Iowa ($685), South Dakota ($785), and Vermont ($670).

For osteopathic physicians, the National Board of Osteopathic Medical Examiners (NBOME) administers the Comprehensive Osteopathic Medical Licensing Examination (COMLEX-USA) at various sites throughout the United States. The Level 3 examination fee is $595.

In addition to these USMLE and COMLEX examination fees, most jurisdictions charge processing, application, and administrative fees, ranging from $35 (Pennsylvania DO) to $840 (Alaska); the average is $331. Including these fees, the average total cost of licensure by examination is $976.

Fees for licensure by endorsement, *including processing, application, and administrative fees*, range from $20 in Pennsylvania to $1,295 in California; the average is $371.

The majority of boards require physicians licensed in the state to reregister (or renew) their licenses every 1 or 2 years; five jurisdictions—Illinois, Michigan, Michigan DO, New Mexico, and Puerto Rico—have a 3-year reregistration interval. The reregistration fee ranges from $790 per year in California to $50 per year (Washington DO); the average reregistration fee is $319 per year. Many states offer reduced fees for reregistration of inactive licenses (see Table 19 for more information).

Completion and reporting of a specified number of hours of continuing medical education (CME) is required for reregistration in 54 jurisdictions.

Additional Notes for Specific Licensing Jurisdictions

California—Endorsement fee includes a $442 processing fee, $63 fingerprinting fee, and $790 licensing fee. Resident physician applicants are charged a reduced licensing fee of $395.

Illinois—Reregistration fee for nonresidents is $600. Penalty of $100 is charged if renewal is not submitted by July 31 in the year of renewal.

Ohio—The Federation Credentials Verification Service (FCVS) is required of all physicians applying for Ohio licensure by either examination or endorsement. The applicable FCVS fee is in addition to the application fee paid to the medical board.

Table 15
Licensure, Endorsement, and Reregistration Fees and Intervals; CME Reporting Requirements

	Examination							Licensure Reregistration			
	USMLE Step 3 Fee ($)	COMLEX Level 3 Fee ($)	Other Application Fees ($)	Total Cost ($)	Application to: FSMB	Application to: NBOME	Endorsement Fees ($)	Registration Interval	Regular Fee ($)	CME Reporting Required	Notes
Alabama	655		175	830	No		175	1 yr	200	Yes	
Alaska	655		840	1,495	Yes		250	2 yrs	590	Yes	$250: Application fee for licensure endorsement
Arizona	655		500	1,155	Yes		500	2 yrs	500	Yes	
Arizona DO		595	400	995		Yes		2 yrs	636	Yes	Biennial fee
Arkansas	655		400	1,055	Yes		400	1 yr	195	Yes	$100 processing fee
California*	655		505	1,160	Yes		1,295	2 yrs	790	Yes	Biennial fee
California DO		595	505	1,100		Yes	256	2 yrs	400	Yes	
Colorado	655		425	1,080	Yes		425	2 yrs	305		
Connecticut	655		450	1,105	Yes		450	1 yr	450		
Delaware	655		0	655	Yes			2 yrs	235	Yes	
DC	655		221	876	No		234	2 yrs	312		
Florida	655		815	1,470	Yes		500	2 yrs	355	Yes	$500 application fee for licensure
Florida DO		595	605	1,200		Yes		2 yrs	405	Yes	
Georgia	655		400	1,055	Yes		400	2 yrs	150	Yes	
Guam	655		400	1,055	Yes		400	2 yrs	250	Yes	
Hawaii	655		290	945	Yes		290	2 yrs	240	Yes	
Hawaii DO		595	400	995		Yes	400	2 yrs	190		
Idaho	655		0	655	Yes		400	1 or 2 yrs	200	Yes	Reregistration $200/yr
Illinois*	655		300	955	No		300	3 yrs	300	Yes	$300 reregistration in state; $600 out of state
Indiana	655		250	905	Yes		250	2 yrs	200		
Iowa	685		50	735	Yes		496	2 yrs	400	Yes	Online renewal $400; paper renewal $500
Kansas	655		300	955	Yes		300	1 yr	230	Yes	
Kentucky	655		0	655	Yes		250	1 yr	125	Yes	
Louisiana	655		0	655	Yes		382	1 yr	232	Yes	$50 fingerprint fee
Maine	655		450	1,105	Yes		450	2 yrs	400	Yes	
Maine DO		595	350	945		Yes	350	2 yrs	500	Yes	
Maryland	655		790	1,445	Yes		817	2 yrs	513	Yes	Endorsement/initial license $917 for IMGs; Reinstatement of lapsed license: $634 US grads; $734 IMGs
Massachusetts	655		600	1,255	Yes		600	2 yrs	400	Yes	
Michigan	655		150	805	Yes		150	3 yrs	285	Yes	
Michigan DO		595	150	745		Yes	150	3 yrs	285	Yes	
Minnesota	655		200	855	Yes		200	1 yr	192	Yes	
Mississippi	655		500	1,155	Yes		500	1 yr	175	Yes	$150 if renewed online
Missouri	655		300	955	No		300	1 yr	135	Yes	
Montana	655		325	980	Yes		325	1 yr	200		
Nebraska	655		202	857	Yes		202	2 yrs	77	Yes	

(continued on next page)

Table 15 (continued)
Licensure, Endorsement, and Reregistration Fees and Intervals; CME Reporting Requirements

	Examination							Licensure Reregistration			
	USMLE Step 3 Fee ($)	COMLEX Level 3 Fee ($)	Other Application Fees ($)	Total Cost ($)	Application to: FSMB	Application to: NBOME	Endorsement Fees ($)	Registration Interval	Regular Fee ($)	CME Reporting Required	Notes
Nevada	655		600	1,255	Yes		600	2 yrs	600	Yes	$75 criminal background investigation fee
Nevada DO		595	800	1,395		Yes	0	1 yr	400	Yes	
New Hampshire	655		250	905	Yes		250	2 yrs	300	Yes	
New Jersey	655		225	880	Yes		225	2 yrs	580		
New Mexico	655		350	1,005	Yes		350	3 yrs	400	Yes	
New Mexico DO		595	300	895		Yes	300	1 yr	100	Yes	
New York	655		735	1,390	Yes		735	2 yrs	600		
North Carolina	655		350	1,005	Yes		350	1 yr	175	Yes	$20 late fee if registration is > 30 days after birthday
North Dakota	655		200	855	Yes		200	1 yr	150	Yes	
Ohio*	655		335*	990	Yes	Yes	335*	2 yrs	305	Yes	* FCVS fee additional
Oklahoma	655		400	1,055	Yes		400	1 yr	150	Yes	
Oklahoma DO		595	0	595		Yes	400	1 yr	200	Yes	$100 late fee
Oregon	655		350	1,005	Yes		350	2 yrs	420		$150 late fee
Pennsylvania	655		35	690	Yes		20	2 yrs	360	Yes	Endorsement is $80 for IMGs
Pennsylvania DO		595	215	810		Yes		2 yrs	440		
Puerto Rico	655		0	655	No		200	3 yrs	75	Yes	
Rhode Island	655		437	1,092	Yes		437	2 yrs	500	Yes	$100 CSR fee
South Carolina	655		0	655	Yes		600	2 yrs	160	Yes	
South Dakota	785		200	985	Yes		200	1 yr	200		$400 late fee ($200 reinstatement plus $200 renewal)
Tennessee	655		400	1,055	Yes		235	2 yrs	235		$280 out-of-state and international application processing fee (nonrefundable)
Tennessee DO		595	400	995		Yes		2 yrs	285	Yes	
Texas	655		80	735	Yes		805	1 yr	752	Yes	
Utah	655		200	855	Yes	Yes	200	2 yrs	183	Yes	$20 late fee; $50 reinstatement fee (FCVS required)
Vermont	670		350	1,020	Yes		450	2 yrs	400		$25 late fee
Vermont DO		595	500	1,095		Yes	500	2 yrs	500	Yes	
Virgin Islands	NA	NA	NA	NA	NA		NA	1 yr	500	Yes	
Virginia	655		0	655	Yes		302	2 yrs	337	Yes	
Washington	655		300	955	Yes		300	2 yrs	450	Yes	Add $25 for initial license endorsement

Table 15 (continued)
Licensure, Endorsement, and Reregistration Fees and Intervals; CME Reporting Requirements

	Examination							Licensure Reregistration			
	USMLE Step 3 Fee ($)	COMLEX Level 3 Fee ($)	Other Application Fees ($)	Total Cost ($)	Application to: FSMB	Application to: NBOME	Endorsement Fees ($)	Registration Interval	Regular Fee ($)	CME Reporting Required	Notes
Washington DO		595	650	1,245		Yes	650	1 yr	50	Yes	Add $25 for substance abuse monitoring prgm
West Virginia	655		600	1,255	Yes		300	2 yrs	300	Yes	
West Virginia DO		595	200	795		Yes	200	2 yrs	200	Yes	
Wisconsin	655		110	765	No		110	2 yrs	106	Yes	Initial $15 contract fee for USMLE Exam
Wyoming	655		450	1,105	Yes		450	1 yr	200		
Total/Average	**655**	**595**	**331**	**976**	**47**	**16**	**371**		**319**	**54**	

Abbreviations

CME—continuing medical education

FSMB—Federation of State Medical Boards

IMG—international medical graduate

USMLE—United States Medical Licensing Examination

* Refer to introductory text to this table for more information on this state's regulations.

Note: ***All information should be verified with the licensing board; medical licenses are granted to those physicians meeting all state requirements—at the discretion of the board.***

Continuing Medical Education for Licensure Reregistration

Sixty boards (including Wyoming, as of January 1, 2007) require an average of anywhere from 12 hours (Alabama) to 50 hours (several states) of continuing medical education (CME) per year for license reregistration. Some states also mandate CME content, such as HIV/AIDS, risk management, or end of life palliative care. In addition, many states also require that a certain percentage of CME be category 1, as measured, for example, through the American Medical Association Physician's Recognition Award. Forty-seven states accept the AMA PRA certificate as equivalent for purposes of licensure reregistration.

Additional Notes for Specific Licensing Jurisdictions

California—All general internists and family physicians who have a patient population of which more than 25% are 65 years of age or older shall complete at least 20% of all mandatory continuing education hours in geriatric medicine or the care of older patients.

All physicians and surgeons shall complete mandatory continuing education in the subjects of pain management and the treatment of terminally ill and dying patients (one-time requirement of 12 credit hours, to be completed by December 31, 2006). Physicians practicing in pathology or radiology specialty areas are exempt from this requirement.

Florida—Physicians may complete a 1-hour CME course on end-of-life and palliative health care in lieu of the required 1-hour CME course on HIV/AIDS, provided the physician completed the HIV/AIDS course in the immediately preceding biennium (2-year licensure term).

Physicians may complete a 1-hour CME course on end-of-life and palliative health care in lieu of the required 1-hour CME course on domestic violence, provided the physician completed the domestic violence course in the immediately preceding biennium (2-year licensure term).

Maryland—Partial CME credit is offered for American Board of Medical Specialties (ABMS) certification, select peer review, serving as an intervenor or monitor on a physician rehabilitation committee or professional committee, and serving as a preceptor for resident physicians or medical students in LCME-accredited schools. For first license renewal, the CME requirement is waived, but the licensee must have completed an approved orientation program.

Washington Osteopathic—Other certificates accepted as equivalent include current certification of CME from medical practice academies and original certification or recertification within 6 years by a specialty board.

Table 16
Continuing Medical Education for Licensure Reregistration

	Required Number of CME Hours per Year(s)		Average Hours per Year	AMA/AOA/AAFP/ACOG Category 1 Hours Required	Certificates Accepted as Equivalent	State-Mandated CME Content/ Additional Notes
Alabama	24 hrs	2 yrs	12	24	ACOG, AAFP	
Alaska	50 hrs	2 yrs	25	25	AMA PRA, ABMS, AOA, APA	
Arizona	40 hrs	2 yrs	20		AMA PRA application, ABMS, GME	40 hrs within 2-yr timeframe
Arizona DO	40 hrs	2 yrs	20	20	AMA PRA	Category 1-A only
Arkansas	20 hrs	1 yr	20	20	AMA PRA	
California*	100 hrs	4 yrs	25	100	AMA PRA, AAFP, CMA, CAFP	Pain management/geriatric medicine (see note)
California DO	150 hrs	3 yrs	50	90	AAFP, CMA, CAFP, AOA	60 hrs Category 1-A or 1-B pain management/geriatric med
Colorado	none					
Connecticut	50 hrs	2 yrs	25			1 hr in infectious disease
Delaware	40 hrs	2 yrs	20	40	AMA PRA, AOA	
DC	50 hrs	2 yrs	25	50	AMA PRA	
Florida*	40 hrs	2 yrs	20	40	AMA PRA	HIV/AIDS, domestic violence, TB, end of life palliative care, med error
Florida DO	40 hrs	2 yrs	20	20 (AOA Category 1-A)		HIV/AIDS, domestic violence, risk management, FL rules/laws, use/abuse of controlled substances, 2 hrs prevention of medical errors
Georgia	40 hrs	2 yrs	20	40	AMA PRA, AOA, AAFP, ACOG, ACEP	
Guam	100 hrs	2 yrs	50	50	AMA PRA, AOA, AAFP, ACOG, ACEP	
Hawaii	40 hrs	2 yrs	20	40	AMA PRA	
Hawaii DO	none					
Idaho	40 hrs	2 yrs	20	40	AMA PRA, ABMS, AOA	
Illinois	150 hrs	3 yrs	50	60	AMA PRA, AOA	
Indiana	none					
Iowa	40 hrs	2 yrs	20	40		Child/dependent adult abuse required every 5 yrs for emergency med, family med, internal med, gen med, ob/gyn, and psych
Kansas	50 hrs	1 yr	50	20	AMA PRA, AAFP, ABMS, GME, AOA	
Kentucky	60 hrs	3 yrs	20	30	AMA PRA, ABMS	One-time domestic violence course for primary care physicans; 2 hrs HIV/AIDS every 10 yrs; course must be approved by Kentucky Cabinet for Hlth Svcs
Louisiana	20 hrs	1 yr	20	20	AMA PRA	One-time board orientation course
Maine	100 hrs	2 yrs	50	40	AMA PRA, ABMS, AAFP	
Maine DO	100 hrs	2 yrs	50	20	AOA	
Maryland*	50 hrs	2 yrs	25	50	AMA PRA application	(see note)
Massachusetts	100 hrs	2 yrs	50	40	AMA PRA, GME	Study board reqs; risk mgmt
Michigan	150 hrs	3 yrs	50	75		
Michigan DO	150 hrs	3 yrs	50	60		60 hrs Category 1-A or 1-B
Minnesota	75 hrs	3 yrs	25	75	AMA PRA, AOA, MOCOMP	

(continued on next page)

Table 16 (continued)
Continuing Medical Education for Licensure Reregistration

	Required Number of CME Hours per Year(s)		Average Hours per Year	AMA/AOA/AAFP/ACOG Category 1 Hours Required	Certificates Accepted as Equivalent	State-Mandated CME Content/ Additional Notes
Mississippi	40 hrs	2 yrs	20	40	AMA PRA app, ABMS, AOA, AAFP , ACOG	
Missouri	50 hrs	2 yrs	25	50	AAFP	
Montana	none					
Nebraska	50 hrs	2 yrs	25	50	AMA PRA	
Nevada	40 hrs	2 yrs	20	40	AMA PRA	Ethics (2 hrs), 20 hrs in specialty; 18 hrs Category 1
Nevada DO	35 hrs	1 yr	35	10	AMA PRA	
New Hampshire	150 hrs	3 yrs	50	60	AMA PRA, ABMS	Credits reported to NH Med Soc
New Jersey	100 hrs	2 yrs	50	40	AMA PRA, AOA	Cultural competence
New Mexico	75 hrs	3 yrs	25	75	AMA PRA, ABMS, AAFP, ACOG	
New Mexico DO	75 hrs	3 yrs	25	75	AMA PRA, ABMS, AAFP, ACOG, USMLE	Active membership in AOA may replace 75 hours of CME
New York	none					Infection control, child abuse
North Carolina	150 hrs	3 yrs	50	60		
North Dakota	60 hrs	3 yrs	20	60	AMA PRA, AOA, AAFP, MOCOMP	
Ohio	100 hrs	2 yrs	50	40	AMA PRA	CME must be OSMA/OOA-certified
Oklahoma	60 hrs	3 yrs	20	60	AMA PRA, ABMS	
Oklahoma DO	16 hrs	1 yr	16	16		16 hrs of Category 1, 1 hr of which must be CME on prescribing controlled substances (every 2 yrs)
Oregon	none					
Pennsylvania	100 hrs	2 yrs	50	20	AMA PRA application	12 hrs patient safety/risk mgmt
Pennsylvania DO	100 hrs	2 yrs	50	20	AOA	20 hrs Category 1-A AOA; 12 hrs risk management/patient safety
Puerto Rico	60 hrs	3 yrs	20	40	AMA PRA	
Rhode Island	40 hrs	2 yrs	20	40	AMA PRA, AOA	HIV universal precautions/ blood-borne pathogens; end of life education/palliative care
South Carolina	40 hrs	2 yrs	20	40	AMA PRA, ABMS, AOA, ACOG equivalent	
South Dakota	none					
Tennessee	40 hrs	2 yrs	20	40	AMA PRA, AAFP	
Tennessee DO	40 hrs	2 yrs	20	40	AMA PRA, AOA, AAFP	
Texas	24 hrs	1 yr	24	12	AMA PRA, AAFP, AOA	Of 12 hrs Category 1, at least 1 hr in ethics/prof. responsibility
Utah	40 hrs	2 yrs	20	20	AMA PRA	
Vermont	none					
Vermont DO	30 hrs	2 yrs	15		AMA PRA	At least 12 of 30 hrs must be osteopathic med education
Virgin Islands	25 hrs	1 yr	25	25		
Virginia	60 hrs	2 yrs	30	30		Of Category 1, 15 hrs must be interactive

Table 16 (continued)
Continuing Medical Education for Licensure Reregistration

	Required Number of CME Hours per Year(s)		Average Hours per Year	AMA/AOA/AAFP/ACOG Category 1 Hours Required	Certificates Accepted as Equivalent	State-Mandated CME Content/ Additional Notes
Washington	200 hrs	4 yrs	50	80	AMA PRA, ABMS, AAFP, ACOG	
Washington DO*	150 hrs	3 yrs	50	60	AMA PRA, AOA, others (see note)	
West Virginia	50 hrs	2 yrs	25	50	AMA PRA, ABMS (partial)	2 hrs end-of-life pain management (one-time requirement)
West Virginia DO	32 hrs	2 yrs	16	16	Board-recognized equivalent	2 hrs end-of-life pain management prior to first license reregistration
Wisconsin	30 hrs	2 yrs	15	30	AMA PRA	
Wyoming	60 hrs	3 yrs	20	60	AMA PRA	Effective Jan 1, 2007

Abbreviations

ABMS—certification or recertification by a member board of the American Board of Medical Specialties

AMA PRA—American Medical Association Physician's Recognition Award

AOA—American Osteopathic Association

AAFP—American Academy of Family Practice

ACOG—American College of Obstetricians and Gynecologists

APA—American Pediatric Association

CMA—California Medical Association

CAFP—California Academy of Family Physicians

CME—continuing medical education

FLEX—Federation Licensing Examination

GME—graduate medical education

MOCOMP—Royal College of Physicians and Surgeons of Canada

OSMA—Ohio State Medical Association

USMLE—United States Medical Licensing Association

* Refer to introductory text to this table for more information on this state's regulations.

Note: ***All information should be verified with licensing board; medical licenses are granted to those physicians meeting all state requirements—at the discretion of the board.***

Resident/Fellow Physician Licenses

Sixty-one jurisdictions issue educational licenses, permits, certificates, or registration to resident/fellow physicians in graduate medical education (GME) programs, with fees ranging from $0 to $300 per year. (The GME program director generally provides a list of residents/fellows and any other required information directly to the licensing jurisdiction.) In 35 of those jurisdictions, residents/fellows must obtain a new permit/license when changing residency/fellowship programs within the state.

Medical boards in 14 states require that prospective residents have passed United States Medical Licensing Examination (USMLE) Step 1 to receive a permit/license. California, Mississippi, Montana, North Dakota, and Utah require passage of Steps 1 and 2.

Sixteen states require that resident/fellow physicians obtain full licensure (not limited or training licenses) at some point in their training (usually after having completed a certain number of years of GME).

Additional Notes for Specific Licensing Jurisdictions

California—Permits are awarded on an individual basis for a maximum of 5 years to noncitizen physicians for postgraduate work in a California medical school.

IMGs must submit an application to determine that all core requirements have been met before they may begin training in California.

Illinois—Limited temporary licenses (valid for 6 months) are awarded to persons in non-Illinois residency programs who are accepted for a specific period of time to perform a portion of that program at a clinical residency program in Illinois due to the lack of adequate facilities in their state.

Visiting Resident Permits are issued for 180 days to persons who have been invited or appointed for a specific period of time to perform a portion of that clinical residency program under the supervision of an Illinois-licensed physician in an Illinois patient care clinic or facility affiliated with the out-of-state GME program.

Massachusetts—Limited registration is issued to physicians enrolled in accredited residency programs and physicians enrolled in fellowships at hospitals with accredited residency programs in the area of the applicant's specialty.

Mississippi—Institutional license is issued to interns and IMG physicians providing health care in state institutions. Applicants are not required to meet all requirements for permanent unrestricted licensure.

Restricted temporary license is issued to physicians enrolled in first year of GME at the University of Mississippi School of Medicine for practice limited to that school.

Addictionology Fellowship License is issued to physicians admitted for treatment in a board-approved drug and/or alcohol addiction treatment program or to physicians enrolled in fellowship of addictionology of the Mississippi State Medical Association Impaired Professionals Program.

Oregon—Limited license (LL) is issued for SPEX, Special, Postgraduate (PG), and Fellow. LL Fellow licenses may be renewed for 1 additional year, LL-PG annually until training is completed.

Pennsylvania—Interim Limited License (up to 12 consecutive months) is issued to physicians providing medical service other than at the training location of the licensee's accredited GME program.

Graduate License allows the licensee to participate for a period of up to 12 consecutive months in GME within the complex of the hospital to which the licensee is assigned and any satellite facility or other training location used in the program.

South Dakota—Resident physicians practicing within the confines of their residency program are not required to obtain a certificate from the board.

A resident physician who wishes to practice on an irregular basis outside their program may apply for a resident certificate if they have completed at least 1 year of GME and remain enrolled in good standing in their program until successful completion. To apply for this certificate, they must meet South Dakota's examination requirements for completion of the entire USMLE within a 7-year period and passing of each step within three attempts. The fee for this certificate is $50.

Table 17
Resident/Fellow Physician Licenses

	Licenses, Permits, Certificates, & Registration	Must Obtain New Permit/License When Changing Residency Programs Within State	Prospective Residents Applying for License Must Have Passed USMLE Step 1	Full licensure required at any point during training?	Notes
Alabama					Limited license for residency education only
Alaska	Yes				Residency permits for up to 18 mos to physicians in accredited residency programs in the US
Arizona	Yes, $50/yr	Yes	Yes		Education Training Permit, granted for 5 days.
Arizona DO	Yes	Yes			Education Training Permit, granted for 5 days, $106
Arkansas					Education license must be renewed annually
California*	Yes		Yes (and Step 2)	Yes; after 2 yrs (3 yrs for IMGs)	
California DO				Yes	No CME required
Colorado	Yes, $10	Yes			Training license valid for duration of program; renews every 3 yrs
Connecticut	Yes, $0	Yes			
Delaware	Yes, $0	Yes			
DC				Yes	
Florida*	Yes, $200	Yes			
Florida DO	Yes, $100	Yes			Unlicensed registration number (for interns, residents, and fellows)
Georgia	Yes, $100				Board must be notified of resident changing program within state.
Guam	Yes	Yes	Yes	Yes; after 3 yrs	
Hawaii	Yes, $75				
Hawaii DO	Yes, $75				
Idaho	Yes, $10	Yes		Yes (see note)	After 1 yr GME (US/Canadian graduates), 3 yrs GME (IMGs)
Illinois*	Yes	Yes			
Indiana	Yes, $100	Yes	Yes		Resident permit good for 1 yr, may be renewed annually
Iowa	Yes, $146	Yes			Resident physician license for GME in board-approved pgm under supervision of licensed physician. Issued for full length of pgm.
Kansas	Yes, $40	Yes			
Kentucky	Yes, $75		Yes		Institutional Practice Limited License or Residency Training License to physicians beyond first year of GME while still in training
Louisiana	Yes, $25	Yes			Intern registration for first 12 mos of GME after completing medical school
Maine	Yes, $100	Yes	Yes		Educational permits for 1 yr in a specific training program, renewable for 5 yrs
Maine DO	Yes, $200	Yes			Temp. educational permits for 1 yr in a specific training pgm only
Maryland	Yes, $100	Yes			Registration of med school grads in GME programs
Massachusetts*	Yes, $100	Yes	Yes	Yes; after 7 yrs	
Michigan	Yes, $170	Yes		Yes; after 6 yrs	Limited annual license for up to 6 yrs for GME, renewable each year; includes controlled substance license
Michigan DO	Yes, $170	Yes		Yes; after 6 yrs	Limited annual license for up to 6 yrs for GME; Includes controlled substance license
Minnesota	Yes	Yes			

(continued on next page)

Table 17 (continued)
Resident/Fellow Physician Licenses

	Licenses, Permits, Certificates, & Registration	Must Obtain New Permit/License When Changing Residency Programs Within State	Prospective Residents Applying for License Must Have Passed USMLE Step 1	Full licensure required at any point during training?	Notes
Mississippi*	Yes, $50/$200		Yes (and Step 2)	Yes; after 5 yrs	
Missouri	Yes, $30	Yes			Temporary licenses issued to interns, residents, and fellows only
Montana	Yes, $100/$50		Yes (and Step 2)		Refer to 37-3-305, MCA
Nebraska	Yes, $25	Yes		Yes; after 5 yrs	Temporary educational permits for residents
Nevada	Yes, $375	Yes		Yes (see note)	Limited 1-yr license for clinical residents ($250 initial, $50 renewal, $75 criminal background investigation). Full licensure usually for fellows/chief residents; depends on program needs
Nevada DO	Yes, $200	Yes			
New Hampshire	Yes, $150	Yes	Yes		
New Jersey	Yes, $50	Yes		Yes; after 5 yrs	Residency training permit required for unlicensed residents in GY2+
New Mexico	Yes, $10		Yes		
New Mexico DO	Yes, $25				
New York	Yes, $105				Requires limited permit for all medical school graduates except individuals in ACGME- or AOA-accredited residency programs. Requires ECFMG certificate from all IMGs for limited permit.
North Carolina	Yes, $100 (permit); $125 (registration)	Yes			Limited license to resident physicians (ineligible for licensure by endorsement)
North Dakota	Yes, $25		Yes (and Step 2)		Limited license for residents in clinical program, renewable annually
Ohio	Yes, $75 (initial) $35 (renewal)	Yes		Yes; after 6 yrs	Training certificate or full license mandatory for interns, residents, and clinical fellows.
Oklahoma	Yes, $200	Yes	Yes		
Oklahoma DO	NA				
Oregon*	Yes, $175	Yes			
Pennsylvania*	Yes, $30				Graduate license renewal fee is $15
Pennsylvania DO	Yes, $30	Yes			Temporary license for GME valid for up to 12 mos; renewal fee $25
Puerto Rico	Yes				Internship/residency licenses to qualified applicants enrolled in an ACGME-accredited residency program who have successfully completed the first part of the medical board examination (basic sciences) or its equivalent (NBME, FLEX, or USMLE)
Rhode Island	Yes, $25	Yes		Yes; after 5 yrs	Limited medical registration to interns, residents, or fellows. Practice limited to the designated institution and must be under the supervision of a staff physician licensed in RI.
South Carolina	Yes, $150	Yes			Limited licenses for residency programs or limited practices renewable on a yearly basis
South Dakota*					(See note)
Tennessee	Yes, $25	Yes			
Tennessee DO	Yes, $50				
Texas	Yes, $144	Yes			

Table 17 (continued)
Resident/Fellow Physician Licenses

	Licenses, Permits, Certificates, & Registration	Must Obtain New Permit/License When Changing Residency Programs Within State	Prospective Residents Applying for License Must Have Passed USMLE Step 1	Full licensure required at any point during training?	Notes
Utah	Yes, $200		Yes (and Step 2)		
Vermont	Yes, $50				Limited license to interns, residents, fellows, or house officers enrolled in ACGME-accredited residency programs and working under supervision of licensed physician at a state-licensed institution or clinic
Vermont DO	Yes, $50				
Virgin Islands	Yes				For residents, institutional license only
Virginia	Yes, $55				Limited license for fellowship and teaching positions. Temporary licenses (renewable annually) to interns, residents, and fellows in accredited programs in Virginia
Washington	Yes, $225				Limited license to physicians in GME and teaching/research at state institutions and city/county health departments
Washington DO	Yes, $300				Limited licensure for GME only
West Virginia					
West Virginia DO	Yes, $50			Yes; after 1 yr	1-yr limited medical registration for interns
Wisconsin	Yes, $10			Yes; after 4 yrs	Temporary educational certificates for residency education after first year
Wyoming	Yes, $25			Yes; after 1 yr	
Total	**61**	**36**	**14**	**16**	

* Refer to introductory text to this table for more information on this state's regulations.

Note: ***All information should be verified with licensing board; medical licenses are granted to those physicians meeting all state requirements—at the discretion of the board.***

Resident/Fellow Physician Licenses: Documentation and Verification

Each state has varying requirements as to the documentation sent to teaching hospitals and/or residents/fellows for those physicians who have a limited educational license for the purposes of graduate education. Wall certificates, wallet cards, and letters are three commonly used forms of documentation.

In addition, most boards maintain archival records of resident/fellow licenses, for varying periods of time, and 44 boards will provide these records to other state boards for licensing/ credentialing purposes.

Table 18
Resident/Fellow Physician Licenses: Documentation and Verification

	Documentation that resident/fellow physicians receive with their license information	Verification of the resident/fellow license is provided to other state boards	Length of time resident/fellow license records are maintained
Alabama		Not applicable	—
Alaska	Permit only	Yes	
Arizona	Wallet card	Yes	Since 1964
Arizona DO	Wall certificate; wallet card	Yes	5 yrs
Arkansas	Letter and registration card; later a wall certificate	—	—
California			
California DO	Wall certificate; wallet card	Yes	
Colorado	License	Yes	Indefinitely
Connecticut	None	No	—
Delaware	License sent to hospital	Yes	30 yrs
DC	Letter to program; posted on Web	Yes	2 yrs
Florida	Letter	Yes	
Florida DO	Letter to resident/fellow and letter to program		
Georgia	Wallet card	Yes	Since 2004
Guam	Primary verification		
Hawaii	Wall certificate, pocket ID	Yes	10 yrs
Hawaii DO			
Idaho	Wall certificate	Yes	14 yrs
Illinois	Letter to program; printed license with program name	Yes	Indefinitely
Indiana	Wall certificate	Yes	Indefinitely
Iowa	Letter sent to resident and program	Yes	10 yrs
Kansas	Wall certificate	Yes	Indefinitely
Kentucky	Letter	Yes	Indefinitely
Louisiana	Wall certificate, letter, orientation info, DEA info	Yes	
Maine	Wall certificate, to the program	Yes	Indefinitely
Maine DO			
Maryland	—	Yes	4 yrs
Massachusetts	Certificate and wallet card	Yes	10 yrs
Michigan	License only; info on purchasing wall certificate	Yes	15 yrs
Michigan DO	License only; info on purchasing wall certificate	Yes	15 yrs
Minnesota	Letter	Yes	Since 1940
Mississippi	Wall certificate and letter	Yes	Indefinitely
Missouri	Wall certificate	Yes	Indefinitely
Montana	Temporary license	Yes	Since January 2004
Nebraska	License card and letter	Yes	Indefinitely
Nevada	Wallet card	Yes	30-plus yrs
Nevada DO			
New Hampshire	Letter	Yes	

(continued on next page)

Table 18 (continued)
Resident/Fellow Physician Licenses: Documentation and Verification

	Documentation that resident/fellow physicians receive with their license information	Verification of the resident/fellow license is provided to other state boards	Length of time resident/fellow license records are maintained
New Jersey	Training permit to pgm	Yes (only to confirm that a training permit was issued; no verification of "standing")	
New Mexico	Certifiate sent to program	Yes	Since 1988
New Mexico DO	Wall certificate, letter, and wallet certificate	Yes	Since 1992
New York			
North Carolina	Certificate	Yes	Indefinitely
North Dakota	Letter with informal certificate	Yes	Since 2001
Ohio	letter to the program	Yes	Since 1999
Oklahoma	Wall certificate, wallet card		
Oklahoma DO			
Oregon	Certificate of registration		
Pennsylvania	Wallet card, 5x7 certificate sent to program	Yes	
Pennsylvania DO	Training permit/registration to hospital		
Puerto Rico			
Rhode Island		Yes	25 yrs
South Carolina	Wallet card	Yes	Since 2003
South Dakota	n/a	n/a	
Tennessee	None	Yes	Indefinitely
Tennessee DO			
Texas	Letter to program	Yes	Records on computer since mid-1980s
Utah	Wall certificate (available for purchase)	n/a	
Vermont	Hardcopy of license	Yes	20 yrs
Vermont DO			
Virgin Islands	n/a	n/a	
Virginia	License renewal certificate	Yes	Indefinitely
Washington	Wall certificate to program only	Yes	Indefinitely
Washington DO	Letter	Yes	75 yrs
West Virginia	Resident/training license not issued	n/a	
West Virginia DO	Letter, wall certificate (if requested)		
Wisconsin	Wall certificate	Yes	
Wyoming	Wall certificate, wallet card	Yes	As of July 1, 2006
Total		**44**	

Note: ***All information should be verified with licensing board; medical licenses are granted to those physicians meeting all state requirements—at the discretion of the board.***

Noneducational Temporary or Limited Licenses, Permits, Certificates, and Registration

Fifty-two boards issue noneducational temporary permits, limited and temporary licenses, or other certificates for the practice of medicine, with fees ranging from $0 to $300 (Maine). The terms for the issuance of such certificates vary, but in general they must be renewed once a year with a stipulated maximum number of renewals allowed (usually 5 years). Often, a board will issue a temporary license or permit valid until the next board meeting, at which a candidate's application will be considered.

Some states permit state institutions to hire unlicensed physicians to work under the supervision of licensed physicians. In many instances, the state departments of mental health and public health that operate these hospitals will not hire physicians who have not had at least 1 year of GME in an English-speaking hospital. International medical graduates are generally not considered for these positions unless they are in the United States with a permanent resident visa. An unlicensed physician employed by a state hospital is required in most states to register with the state board of medical examiners, which may issue a limited permit to practice within the institution.

Fourteen jurisdictions issue locum tenens permits, with fees ranging from $0 to $525 (Nevada MD board).

Thirty jurisdictions issue inactive licenses (for physicians who want to maintain licensure in that state although they are currently practicing in another state), with fees ranging from $0 to $420 (Oregon).

Seventeen jurisdictions issue retired physicians' licenses, with fees ranging from $0 to $200 (Nevada DO board), and 13 issue camp licenses.

Table 19
Noneducational Temporary or Limited Licenses, Permits, Certificates, and Registration

	Noneducational Temporary/Limited Licenses, Permits, and Certificates	Locum Tenens Permits	Inactive Licenses	Retired Physicians' Licenses	Camp Licenses	Additional Notes
Alabama	Yes, $175					Limited license for work in penal and mental institutions
Alaska*	Yes, $145	Yes	Yes, $225	Yes, $50		Retired physician license: $50 one-time fee
Arizona*	Yes	Yes, $350				
Arizona DO	Yes	Yes, $300				
Arkansas*	Yes, $50					
California*			Yes	Yes, $0		
California DO			Yes, $150			
Colorado			Yes			
Connecticut	Yes, $150					Temporary permits (valid for 1 year only, not renewable or extendable) only to those physicians who have been offered a position in a state hospital or state facility
Delaware						
DC			Yes, $312			
Florida*	Yes (See note)		Yes, $55			
Florida DO	Yes, $100		Yes, $100	Yes, $55		
Georgia	Yes, $100		Yes, $140			Temporary permits for reciprocity/endorsement applicants between board meetings
Guam	Yes, $275		Yes, $300			Temporary permits for reciprocity/endorsement applicants between board meetings
Hawaii*	Yes					Not available to physicians against whom disciplinary action is pending in another state
Idaho	Yes, $100		Yes, $75	Yes		Temporary license while awaiting criminal background check outcome; clear routine applicants only; all requirements met; complete application required; good for 120 days. May be extended by board order. Inactive license holders may not practice or prescribe. Volunteer license to retired physicians for uncompensated practice (no fee).
Illinois*	Yes		Yes			
Indiana*	Yes, $100	Yes, $100	Yes, $100	Yes, $100	Yes, $100	Inactive/retired lic are same status. Camp lic limited scope
Iowa	Yes, $246					Temporary license for urgent need
Kansas*	Yes, $40		Yes, $115	Yes, $130		Physicians with inactive licenses may not practice medicine in any form, including writing prescriptions.
Kentucky*	Yes					Temporary permit until board meets (for endorsement candidates only)
Louisiana*	Yes, $0			Yes, $100		
Maine	Yes, $300	Yes		Yes	Yes, $100	Retired physicians' license for those doing volunteer work; volunteer license is $75; temporary and camp licenses (up to 1 yr) for duration of community need
Maine DO	Yes	Yes, $200			Yes, $100	
Maryland	Yes, $100		Yes, $50			Physicians with inactive licenses may not practice medicine in any form, including writing prescriptions. Residents must register with the board annually.
Massachusetts		Yes				

Table 19 (continued)
Noneducational Temporary or Limited Licenses, Permits, Certificates, and Registration

	Noneducational Temporary/Limited Licenses, Permits, and Certificates	Locum Tenens Permits	Inactive Licenses	Retired Physicians' Licenses	Camp Licenses	Additional Notes
Michigan				Yes, $0		For practice in underserved areas, with no remuneration; reviewed annually
Michigan DO				Yes, $0		For practice in underserved areas, with no remuneration; reviewed annually
Minnesota	Yes, $60			Yes, $50	Yes, $0	Temporary license valid until next board meeting at which application is to be considered
Mississippi	Yes				Yes, $25	Ninety-day Youth Camp Permit issued to physicians providing health care only at youth camps approved by the Mississippi State Department of Health
Missouri	No			Yes, $25		
Montana*	Yes, $325		Yes, $100	Yes, $32.50		Additional $325 for temporary permit
Nebraska*		Yes, $101	Yes, $25			
Nevada	Yes	Yes, $525	Yes, $300 (every 2 yrs)			Locum tenens license (one-time only) for 3 months to qualified candidates. Temporary licenses for practice in medically underserved areas (at discretion of the board). $75 criminal background investigation fee.
Nevada DO	Yes, $200		Yes, $200			
New Hampshire*	Yes, $150	Yes, $150			Yes, $75	
New Jersey*	Yes			Yes, $125		
New Mexico	Yes, $100		Yes		Yes, $25	
New Mexico DO	Yes, $0					Issued to physicians who have applied for and met licensure requirements between regular board meetings
New York	Yes					
North Carolina	Yes, $150		Yes		Yes, $100	Limited license for practice in medically underserved areas; temporary licenses to eligible endorsement candidates beginning practice prior to board meeting
North Dakota*	Yes, $200	Yes, $200		Yes		Locum tenens permit not to exceed 3 months; no fee for lifetime special emeritus license status (may not practice)
Ohio*	Yes		Yes, $0 volunteer certificate	Yes, $0 Emeritus certificate		Limited certificates for employment in state hospitals. Retired physician license. Special activity certificate $125.
Oklahoma*	Yes			Yes		Emeritus (may not practice); limited volunteer license for uncompensated practice
Oklahoma DO	NA					
Oregon*	Yes, $175		Yes, $420		Yes, $420	Locum tenens license limited to 180 days' practice in state in the biennium
Pennsylvania*	Yes			Yes		
Pennsylvania DO	Yes			Yes	Yes, $45	
Puerto Rico*	Yes					
Rhode Island	Yes		Yes, $0			Emeritus status (inactive license)
South Carolina	Yes, $75		Yes, $0			Temporary license to any applicant who meets all requirements pending final board approval

(continued on next page)

Table 19 (continued)
Noneducational Temporary or Limited Licenses, Permits, Certificates, and Registration

	Noneducational Temporary/Limited Licenses, Permits, and Certificates	Locum Tenens Permits	Inactive Licenses	Retired Physicians' Licenses	Camp Licenses	Additional Notes
South Dakota		Yes, $50				Sixty-day locum tenens permit
Tennessee	Yes	Yes	Yes, $50			
Tennessee DO			Yes, $50			
Texas	Yes, $50					Temporary licenses pending final board approval
Utah			Yes, $50			Inactive license must be renewed every 2 yrs; $50 to make active again
Vermont						
Vermont DO	Yes					
Virgin Islands	Yes					Temp licenses (2 yrs) for government employment only
Virginia	Yes		Yes, $168		Exemption authorized $25	Temporary license/certificate for continuing education, summer camps, and free clinics
Washington	Yes			Yes		Temporary permit (valid 90 days) only in conjunction with full application; applicant must have been previously licensed in an approved state
Washington DO	Yes		Yes			Must be applicant for a full license; valid for 90 days. Not renewable. Must be licensed and in good standing in another state.
West Virginia	Yes		Yes, $100		Yes	Temporary license (valid until subsequent board meeting) after completed application for permanent license has been filed, processed, and found in order
West Virginia DO	Yes					Temporary license granted, at discretion of board, for specific location and need
Wisconsin	Yes, $135	Yes, $163			Yes	Camp physician license or locum tenens for up to 90 days
Wyoming	Yes, $100			Yes; only if living in state		Temporary license between board meetings after completed application for permanent license has been filed, processed, and approved by the board
Total	**52**	**14**	**30**	**21**	**13**	

* Refer to additional text on following pages for more information on this state's regulations.

Note: ***All information should be verified with licensing board; medical licenses are granted to those physicians meeting all state requirements—at the discretion of the board.***

Table 19 (continued)
Noneducational Temporary or Limited Licenses, Permits, Certificates, and Registration

Alaska
- Temporary permits for specific period (6 months maximum) after completed application is on file and until board meets to consider permanent licensure.
- Locum tenens permit for 90 days to an MD or DO licensed in another state for purpose of substituting for another Alaska-licensed physician; may extend 1-60 days.

Arizona
- Locum tenens permit for a 180-day period to a licensed MD to temporarily assist or substitute for an MD licensed in Arizona.

Arkansas
- Temporary permits for limited time in emergency or hardship cases, only after application for licensure is complete and waiting to be presented to the board. Valid until next board meeting.

Florida
- Temporary Certificate to Practice in Area of Critical Need ($300) to MDs/DOs with current valid license in another state to practice in Florida communities with a critical need for physicians and a population of less than 7,500.
- Limited License ($210) to MDs/DOs who meet the same minimum education and training requirements as required for a full medical license and who are retired and have been licensed to practice medicine in any jurisdiction in the United States for at least 10 years. Practice restricted to public agencies or institutions or nonprofit agencies or institutions meeting the requirements of Section 501(c)(3) of the Internal Revenue Code and located in areas of critical medical need.
- A Public Psychiatry Certificate to board-certified psychiatrists who are licensed to practice medicine without restriction in another state and who meet the minimum education and training requirements required for a full medical license. Practice is restricted to a public mental health facility or program funded in part or entirely by state funds.
- A Public Health Certificate to MDs/DOs who are graduates of an accredited medical/osteopathic school and hold a master of public health degree or are board-eligible or certified in public health or preventive medicine, or to MDs/DOs who are licensed to practice medicine without restriction in another jurisdiction in the United States and hold a master of public health degree or are board eligible or certified in public health or preventive medicine and who meet the minimum education and training requirements required for a full medical/osteopathic license. Practice restricted to employment duties with the Department of Health and Rehabilitative Services.

Hawaii
- Temporary license to physicians working in a state or county agency in conditions of shortage or emergency; and to physicians under the supervision of a licensed MD who plan to take the USMLE exam within 18 months.

Illinois
- Visiting Physician Permits for up to 180 days to persons receiving an invitation or appointment to study, demonstrate, or perform a specific medical, osteopathic, or chiropractic subject or technique in medical, osteopathic, or chiropractic schools; hospitals; or facilities operated pursuant to the Ambulatory Surgical Treatment Center Act.

Indiana
- To physicians holding an active, valid license from another US/Canadian jurisdiction who have applied for and are awaiting board approval of permanent unrestricted license by endorsement of another jurisdiction's valid license; valid for a designated period of 90 days or less.
- To physicians holding a valid, active license from another US/Canadian jurisdiction who are providing health care for a circumscribed period as part of a special program, event, or other activity, including locum tenens; permit valid for up to 30 days and is not renewable.

Kansas
- Temporary permit until next licensure board meeting after application for licensure has been completed, filed, processed, and found to be in order. No temporary permit before passing examination.
- Institutional permits to work in state institutions or mental health centers.
- Out-of-phase special permit.

Kentucky
- Temporary permit until next licensure board meeting after application for licensure has been completed, filed, processed, and found to be in order. No temporary permit before passing examination.

Louisiana
- Unrestricted temporary permits only under extreme circumstances. Board meets every 4 weeks to act on reciprocity licensure applications. Board must act on SPEX applicants requiring unrestricted temporary permit. SPEX applicants issued institutional temporary permit, if necessary, pending results of exam.
- Ninety-day renewable unrestricted permit, pending valid visa issued by the Immigration and Naturalization Service.

Montana
- Temporary license to physicians for practice in specified location in the interval between board meetings. Board may ask physician to appear at next board meeting for temporary license renewal. No requirements are waived.

Nebraska
- Locum tenens permit for a qualified physician with current license in another state for replacement of a Nebraska physician during a period of temporary leave (maximum of 90 days in any 12-month period).

New Hampshire
- Temporary/restricted license, in the state's best interest. Locum tenens (courtesy license) available to a qualified applicant currently holding an unrestricted active license in another state; valid for a maximum of 100 consecutive days in any 12-month period.

New Jersey
- Temporary license (4 months) for a lawfully qualified physician of another state to take charge of the practice of a licensed New Jersey physician during his or her absence from the state. Exemption from licensure to work in county or state institution for a limited period.

North Dakota
- Temporary license between intervals of board meetings; permanent licenses issued only at regularly scheduled meetings (March, July, and November). All licensure requirements must be met and file must be processed completely before a temporary license or locum tenens permit will be issued.

(continued on next page)

Table 19 (continued)
Noneducational Temporary or Limited Licenses, Permits, Certificates, and Registration

Ohio	• Special Activity Certificate ($125) may be issued to qualified applicants seeking to practice in conjunction with a special activity, program, or event taking place in Ohio. The certificate may not be used for locum tenens, is valid for the shorter of 30 days or the duration of the special activity, and cannot be renewed.
Oklahoma	• Temporary medical licenses during the intervals between board meetings. Candidates for temporary license must meet qualifications for full and unrestricted license. Temporary licenses automatically terminate on the date of the next board meeting, when the applicant may be considered for a full and unrestricted medical license.
Oregon	• Limited License SPEX (LL-SPEX) valid while awaiting results of SPEX examination. • Limited License-Special (LL-Special) allows applicant with complete file to practice between two board meetings.
Pennsylvania	• Temporary License allows licensee to participate in a medical procedure necessary for the well-being of a specified patient within the Commonwealth or to practice medicine and surgery at a camp or resort for no more than 3 months. Applicants for a temporary license must hold an unrestricted license in another state, territory, possession, or country. • Extraterritorial License granted to licensed physicians maintaining an office to practice near the boundary line of an adjoining state whose medical practice extends into Pennsylvania.
Puerto Rico	• Public service licenses to qualified applicants who have completed at least 1 year of accredited residency education and who have passed all three parts of the medical board examination or its equivalent (NBME, FLEX, or USMLE).

Note: ***All information should be verified with the licensing board; medical licenses are granted to those physicians meeting all state requirements—at the discretion of the board.***

Regulations on the Practice of Telemedicine and Out-of-state Consulting Physicians

For purposes of this publication, *telemedicine* is defined as the delivery of health care services via electronic means from a health care provider in one location to a patient in another. Applications that fall under this definition include the transfer of medical images, such as pathology slides or radiographs, interactive video consultations between patient and provider or between primary care and specialty care physicians, and mental health consultations. Thirty-two states have adopted regulations concerning the practice of telemedicine; six other states have begun to develop regulations.

Additional Notes for Specific Licensing Jurisdictions

Mississippi—Full license required for physicians rendering a medical opinion concerning diagnosis or treatment via electronic or other means, unless the evaluation, treatment, and/or medical opinion to be rendered by a physician outside this state (a) is requested by a physician duly licensed to practice medicine in this state, and (b) the physician who has requested such evaluation, treatment, and/or medical opinion has already established a doctor/patient relationship with the patient to be evaluated and/or treated.

Table 20
Regulations on the Practice of Telemedicine and Out-of-state Consulting Physicians

	Practice of Telemedicine		
	Has Adopted Regulations	Has Begun to Develop Regulations	Specific Licensure Restrictions on and/or Requirements for Out-of-state Consulting Physicians
Alabama	Yes		Issues a "special purpose" license (1997).
Alaska			Active Alaska license required. Exceptions are made for an MD or DO who is not a resident of Alaska and who is asked by an Alaskan MD or DO to help in the diagnosis or treatment of a case.
Arizona	Yes		No license required for single or infrequent consultation from out-of-state physician with licensed physician. Full license required of any physician providing services via technology.
Arkansas	Yes		
California	Yes		No license required for consultations with a primary care physician licensed in California.
Colorado	Yes		Licensed Colorado physician may consult with physicians licensed in another state. Full license required to use telemedicine to diagnose and treat diseases.
Connecticut	Yes		In the case of electronic transmissions of radiographic images, license required for an out-of-state physician who provides, through an ongoing, regular, or contractual arrangement, official written reports of diagnostic evaluations of such images to Connecticut physicians or patients. No license required of a physician residing outside of Connecticut who, while located outside Connecticut, consults on an irregular basis with a licensed Connecticut physician, who is located in this state, or with a medical school within this state for educational or medical training purposes.
Delaware			No license required, if physician is licensed in another state and performs a consultation no more than 6 times a year.
DC		Yes	
Florida MD and DO	Yes		Physician licensed in another state, territory, or foreign country is permitted to examine the patient, take a history and physical, review laboratory tests and X rays, and make recommendations about diagnosis and treatment to a licensed Florida physician. The term "consultation" does not include such physician's performance of any medical procedure on or the rendering of treatment to the patient. Full licensure required for out-of-state physicians using telemedicine to treat Florida residents.
Georgia	Yes		License required for out-of-state telemedicine.
Guam	Yes		Must hold license in state where physician resides.
Hawaii	Yes		Out-of-state consultant must be licensed in the state in which he/she resides; may not open an office (or appoint a place to meet patients or receive calls) in Hawaii.
Idaho			No license required for out-of-state physicians consulted by licensed Idaho physicians.
Illinois	Yes		Full license required.
Indiana	Yes		
Iowa			No license required for incidental consultation with out-of-state physicians by licensed Iowa physicians; out-of-state physician must be licensed if providing medical services to Iowa patients.
Kansas	Yes		License required if orders for services are issued for individuals located in Kansas. No license required for consultant licensed in another state who does not open an office or maintain a place to meet patients or receive calls in Kansas. No license required for services performed under supervision or by order of or referral from a licensed Kansas physician.
Kentucky	Yes		No license required for single or infrequent consultation from out-of-state physician with licensed physician. Full license required of any physician providing services via technology.
Louisiana			
Maine	Yes		No license required for incidental consultation with out-of-state physicians by licensed Maine physicians; out-of-state physician must be licensed if providing medical services to patients in Maine.
Maryland			Maryland license required, unless in consultation with a licensed Maryland physician and consultation is in Maryland.
Massachusetts			Full license required.
Michigan MD and DO		Yes	No license required for a physician living in and authorized to practice in another state or country who, in exceptional circumstances, is called for consultation or treatment by a Michigan health professional.
Minnesota			Telemedicine registration not required for physicians providing services in response to an emergency condition, services on an irregular or infrequent basis, or services as a consultant with a Minnesota-licensed physician who has ultimate authority over diagnosis and care of patient.
Mississippi	Yes		No license required for out-of-state physicians called for consultation by a licensed physician residing in Mississippi. Consultation period cannot exceed 5 days. Refer to introductory text to this table for more.

Table 20 (continued)
Regulations on the Practice of Telemedicine and Out-of-state Consulting Physicians

	Practice of Telemedicine		
	Has Adopted Regulations	Has Begun to Develop Regulations	Specific Licensure Restrictions on and/or Requirements for Out-of-state Consulting Physicians
Missouri	Yes		Licensed Missouri physician may consult with physicians licensed in another state. Full license required to use telemedicine to diagnose and treat diseases.
Montana	Yes		License required if an out-of-state consultant establishes a regular, direct physician/patient relationship.
Nebraska			Nonresident physicians not holding a Nebraska license cannot practice medicine, except when called in consultation by a licensed Nebraska physician.
Nevada	Yes		Special purpose license required. Active license in home jurisdiction required.
Nevada DO	Yes		Licensure application required.
New Hampshire			License required if consultation is not made directly with a licensed New Hampshire physician or if consulting is more than incidental.
New Jersey		Yes	
New Mexico	Yes		Telemedicine license is required, with some exceptions; contact the Board for more information.
New York		Yes	License in home jurisdiction required.
North Carolina	Yes		North Carolina license required by state law.
North Dakota			North Dakota license required.
Ohio	Yes		Telemedicine license is required, with some exceptions; contact the Board for more information.
Oklahoma	Yes		License required for regular, ongoing treatment; license not required for occasional consultation.
Oregon	Yes		Permanent license required to practice medicine.
Pennsylvania		Yes	Pennsylvania license required.
Puerto Rico			
Rhode Island		Yes	Requirements exist for out-of-state consultants.
South Carolina			Must consult with a licensed South Carolina physician.
South Dakota	Yes		Any nonresident MD or DO who, while located outside South Dakota, provides diagnostic or treatment services through electronic means to a patient in this state under a contract with a health care provider, a clinic in this state that provides health services, or health care facility is engaged in the practice of medicine or osteopathy in South Dakota. Out-of-state MDs or DOs who consult on an irregular basis with a licensed South Dakota physician are not considered to practice in South Dakota.
Tennessee	Yes		Telemedicine license required of out-of-state physicians diagnosing or treating patients in Tennessee. Some exceptions granted.
Texas	Yes		Special Purpose License required for practice of medicine across state lines.
Utah	Yes		No license required of out-of-state physicians consulting with licensed Utah physician; full license required if consulting directly with patient by any means.
Vermont			
Virgin Islands			
Virginia			Virginia license required if practice of medicine occurs in state.
Washington			May not set up an office, appoint a place for meeting patients, or receive calls within this state.
West Virginia	Yes		License required (with exceptions).
West Virginia DO			West Virginia license required.
Wisconsin	Yes		Wisconsin license required.
Wyoming	Yes		No license required of physicians residing in and licensed to practice medicine in another state or country called for consultation via telephone, electronic, or any other means by a licensed Wyoming physician. License required if consultations exceed one 7-day period in any 52-week period.
Total	**32**	**6**	

Note: ***All information should be verified with the licensing board; medical licenses are granted to those physicians meeting all state requirements—at the discretion of the board.***

Section II.

Statistics of State Medical Licensing Boards

Data in this section were taken from the AMA Physician Masterfile, an electronic database that tracks physicians' entire educational and professional careers, from medical school and graduate medical education (GME) through practice. Data include *only* full and unrestricted licenses; limited educational permits or licenses for resident physicians in GME programs are *not* included. Licenses issued to doctors of osteopathy (DOs) are also included.

Please note the following definitions:

Initial License—When a physician without *any* previous licensure receives the first license of his/her professional career.

New License—When a physician without previous licensure from a particular state receives a license from that state.

These two figures overlap, as all initial licenses are a subset of new licenses.

In 2005, 57,184 licenses were issued to doctors of medicine (MDs) and doctors of osteopathy (DOs) by medical licensing boards (see Table 21). Of these, 23,180, or 40.5%, were identified as initial licenses.

Table 22 shows a breakdown of total licenses awarded in 2004 by licensing jurisdiction, by US medical graduates and international medical graduates (IMGs).

Tables 23 through 25 present data on initial licensure. As previously noted, an initial license is the physician's first ever full and unrestricted license.

Table 23 shows the percentage of initial licenses awarded in a given jurisdiction. As previously noted, the national average for 2005 was 40.5%. In the states with higher percentages, then, the physician population is growing more rapidly than the national average.

Table 23 also breaks out the total initial licenses in each state by US medical school graduates and IMGs. Of the 23,180 physicians who received their initial licenses in 2005, 6,789 (29.3%) were issued to IMGs.

Table 21
Licenses Issued to Physicians by State Medical/Osteopathic Boards, 1975–2005

Year	Total New Licenses	Total Initial Licenses
1975	36,621	16,859
1976	38,488	17,724
1977	39,919	18,175
1978	41,457	19,393
1979	42,015	19,896
1980	41,112	18,172
1981	43,092	18,831
1982	43,543	17,605
1983	44,548	20,601
1984	43,681	18,340
1985	41,943	18,288
1986	43,375	19,528
1987	44,998	20,324
1988	44,969	21,235
1989	45,648	20,115
1990	44,341	20,853
1991	45,249	20,962
1992	45,132	19,760
1993	48,834	20,182
1994	49,912	20,857
1995	51,332	22,250
1996	55,716	23,920
1997	55,886	24,151
1998	56,237	23,419
1999	54,586	22,999
2000	51,866	19,581
2001	52,305	21,078
2002	52,877	20,383
2003	52,281	20,632
2004	55,435	22,599
2005	57,184	23,180

Table 24 provides an historical picture of the numbers of initial licenses awarded since 1950 and how the percentages have varied between US medical graduates and IMGs. In 1950, for example, only 5% of initial licensees were IMGs; in 2005, 29% were IMGs. The highest percentage of IMGs as initial licensees occurred in 1972 and 1973, with 46% and 44%, respectively (by 1979, however, the percentage had dropped back to 18%).

Table 23 provides an historical picture of the numbers of IMGs receiving initial licenses by state since 1975.

Table 22
Full Unrestricted Licenses (Whether Physician's Initial or Subsequent) Issued to MDs and DOs by State Medical/Osteopathic Boards, 2005

	Total	US Medical Graduates	IMGs	Percentage of Licenses Awarded to IMGs
Alabama	728	569	159	22
Alaska	391	360	31	8
Arizona	1,464	1,101	363	25
Arkansas	400	294	106	27
California	4,935	3,606	1,329	27
Colorado	970	882	88	9
Connecticut	964	642	322	33
Delaware	316	230	86	27
DC	616	483	133	22
Florida	2,925	1,890	1,035	35
Georgia	1,499	1,101	398	27
Hawaii	416	351	65	16
Idaho	300	277	23	8
Illinois	2,174	1,526	648	30
Indiana	1,650	1,121	529	32
Iowa	585	428	157	27
Kansas	578	448	130	22
Kentucky	809	612	197	24
Louisiana	687	522	165	24
Maine	288	218	70	24
Maryland	1,395	1,045	350	25
Massachusetts	1,774	1,354	420	24
Michigan	1,850	1,152	698	38
Minnesota	960	776	184	19
Mississippi	389	297	92	24
Missouri	1,097	846	251	23
Montana	265	225	40	15
Nebraska	431	361	70	16
Nevada	526	355	171	33
New Hampshire	378	314	64	17
New Jersey	1,759	1,055	704	40
New Mexico	633	471	162	26
New York	3,722	2,473	1,249	34
North Carolina	1,779	1,450	329	18
North Dakota	200	157	43	22
Ohio	2,015	1,441	574	28
Oklahoma	526	394	132	25
Oregon	699	607	92	13
Pennsylvania	2,889	2,128	761	26
Puerto Rico	446	139	307	69
Rhode Island	349	256	93	27
South Carolina	612	486	126	21
South Dakota	172	145	27	16
Tennessee	1,240	985	255	21
Texas	2,551	1,809	742	29
Utah	517	438	79	15
Vermont	196	177	19	10
Virginia	1,858	1,370	488	26
Washington	1,474	1,208	266	18
West Virginia	435	307	128	29
Wisconsin	1,174	873	301	26
Wyoming	178	155	23	13
Total	**57,184**	**41,910**	**15,274**	**27 (avg)**

Table 23
Initial Licenses Issued to MDs and DOs by State Medical/Osteopathic Boards, 2005

	Total	US Medical Graduates	IMGs	Initial Licenses Awarded as Percentage of Full Unrestricted Licenses (Table 20)
Alabama	304	231	73	42
Alaska	26	23	3	7
Arizona	296	216	80	20
Arkansas	127	79	48	32
California	2,888	2,187	701	59
Colorado	273	251	22	28
Connecticut	345	176	169	36
Delaware	66	41	25	21
DC	217	173	44	35
Florida	817	484	333	28
Georgia	353	247	106	24
Hawaii	121	95	26	29
Idaho	24	22	2	8
Illinois	1,162	769	393	53
Indiana	643	415	228	39
Iowa	188	117	71	32
Kansas	196	143	53	34
Kentucky	227	158	69	28
Louisiana	378	281	97	55
Maine	69	42	27	24
Maryland	479	352	127	34
Massachusetts	1,006	759	247	57
Michigan	1,074	600	474	58
Minnesota	456	376	80	48
Mississippi	114	82	32	29
Missouri	396	319	77	36
Montana	15	13	2	6
Nebraska	166	150	16	39
Nevada	69	35	34	13
New Hampshire	79	54	25	21
New Jersey	496	234	262	28
New Mexico	118	63	55	19
New York	2,285	1,561	724	61
North Carolina	528	438	90	30
North Dakota	26	17	9	13
Ohio	1,054	745	309	52
Oklahoma	252	179	73	48
Oregon	167	143	24	24
Pennsylvania	1,554	1,155	399	54
Puerto Rico	410	109	301	92
Rhode Island	101	72	29	29
South Carolina	72	47	25	12
South Dakota	22	15	7	13
Tennessee	370	304	66	30
Texas	1,088	898	190	43
Utah	196	170	26	38
Vermont	41	35	6	21
Virginia	774	539	235	42
Washington	396	313	83	27
West Virginia	142	107	35	33
Wisconsin	501	351	150	43
Wyoming	13	6	7	7
Total	**23,180**	**16,391**	**6,789**	**41 (avg)**

Table 24
Initial Licenses Issued to MDs and DOs by State Medical/Osteopathic Boards, 1950-2005

Year	Total	US Medical Graduates		IMGs	
1950	6,002	5,694	95%	308	5%
1951	6,273	5,923	94%	350	6%
1952	6,885	6,316	92%	569	8%
1953	7,276	6,591	91%	685	9%
1954	7,917	7,145	90%	772	10%
1955	7,737	6,830	88%	907	12%
1956	7,463	6,611	89%	852	11%
1957	7,455	6,441	86%	1,014	14%
1958	7,809	6,643	85%	1,166	15%
1959	8,269	6,643	80%	1,626	20%
1960	8,030	6,611	82%	1,419	18%
1961	8,023	6,443	80%	1,580	20%
1962	8,005	6,648	83%	1,357	17%
1963	8,283	6,832	82%	1,451	18%
1964	7,911	6,605	83%	1,306	17%
1965	9,147	7,619	83%	1,528	17%
1966	8,851	7,217	82%	1,634	18%
1967	9,424	7,343	78%	2,081	22%
1968	9,766	7,581	78%	2,185	22%
1969	9,978	7,671	77%	2,307	23%
1970	11,032	8,016	73%	3,016	27%
1971	12,257	7,943	65%	4,314	35%
1972	14,476	7,815	54%	6,661	46%
1973	16,689	9,270	56%	7,419	44%
1974	16,706	10,093	60%	6,613	40%
1975	16,859	10,794	64%	6,065	36%
1976	17,724	11,288	64%	6,436	36%
1977	18,175	12,324	68%	5,851	32%
1978	19,393	14,815	76%	4,578	24%
1979	19,896	16,330	82%	3,566	18%
1980	18,172	14,862	82%	3,310	18%
1981	18,831	15,700	83%	3,131	17%
1982	17,605	13,409	76%	4,196	24%
1983	20,601	15,848	77%	4,753	23%
1984	18,340	14,246	78%	4,094	22%
1985	18,288	15,239	83%	3,049	17%
1986	19,528	16,592	85%	2,936	15%
1987	20,324	17,096	84%	3,228	16%
1988	21,235	18,005	85%	3,230	15%
1989	20,115	17,366	86%	2,749	14%
1990	20,853	17,254	83%	3,599	17%
1991	20,962	16,959	81%	4,003	19%
1992	19,760	16,008	81%	3,752	19%
1993	20,182	15,805	78%	4,377	22%
1994	20,857	15,961	77%	4,896	23%
1995	22,520	17,201	76%	5,319	24%
1996	23,920	17,486	73%	6,434	27%
1997	24,151	16,714	69%	7,069	31%
1998	23,419	17,786	76%	5,633	24%
1999	22,999	17,700	77%	5,299	23%
2000	19,581	14,586	74%	4,995	26%
2001	21,078	15,392	73%	5,686	27%
2002	20,383	14,888	73%	5,495	27%
2003	20,632	15,019	73%	5,613	27%
2004	22,599	16,239	72%	6,360	28%
2005	23,180	16,391	71%	6,789	29%

Table 25
Initial Licenses Issued to International Medical Graduates by State Medical/Osteopathic Boards, 1975-2005

	1975	1980	1985	1990	1995	2000	2003	2004	2005
Alabama	1	0	8	11	136	28	54	51	73
Alaska	1	0	0	1	15	1	1	13	3
Arizona	20	16	17	14	8	28	63	1	80
Arkansas	8	5	9	13	31	27	46	45	48
California	212	276	243	355	435	392	381	754	701
Colorado	6	6	18	29	6	15	21	24	22
Connecticut	13	54	71	23	11	146	203	176	169
Delaware	9	3	4	9	4	16	14	12	25
DC	426	59	45	19	13	49	52	56	44
Florida	325	114	114	156	155	204	313	342	333
Georgia	74	165	113	38	67	62	114	130	106
Hawaii	14	9	6	15	14	9	12	25	26
Idaho	0	1	0	0	0	1	5	0	2
Illinois	481	94	75	369	631	360	427	411	393
Indiana	46	58	85	50	2	412	274	253	228
Iowa	71	36	132	49	107	73	71	66	71
Kansas	25	23	12	31	122	25	36	47	53
Kentucky	30	30	2	20	38	53	70	72	69
Louisiana	11	21	26	3	35	70	92	101	97
Maine	197	172	3	14	21	11	31	22	27
Maryland	258	244	125	239	213	0	150	132	127
Massachusetts	199	170	42	151	202	208	155	230	247
Michigan	565	146	195	31	431	323	398	474	474
Minnesota	39	16	49	38	50	84	105	115	80
Mississippi	9	5	0	5	0	15	18	33	32
Missouri	124	30	20	16	63	61	83	102	77
Montana	0	4	1	0	3	0	4	1	2
Nebraska	20	30	22	35	5	16	22	14	16
Nevada	5	4	0	1	5	17	32	50	34
New Hampshire	22	4	5	4	38	6	20	12	25
New Jersey	139	262	324	318	321	199	240	186	262
New Mexico	14	11	11	26	7	27	51	49	55
New York	805	594	352	975	640	683	700	835	724
North Carolina	66	19	35	18	57	56	47	50	90
North Dakota	45	20	6	0	6	8	12	20	9
Ohio	183	70	71	43	63	444	203	293	309
Oklahoma	30	72	39	20	25	42	57	70	73
Oregon	14	13	3	6	10	39	21	19	24
Pennsylvania	490	137	253	107	390	342	345	289	399
Puerto Rico	157	4	46	25	97	—	—	2	301
Rhode Island	7	11	20	11	17	30	29	34	29
South Carolina	2	13	1	2	160	20	17	28	25
South Dakota	3	12	5	0	6	3	11	12	7
Tennessee	18	23	20	25	57	48	52	70	66
Texas	201	100	49	54	18	54	127	174	190
Utah	4	1	12	36	237	16	23	18	26
Vermont	46	0	1	3	3	5	10	5	6
Virginia	327	49	43	49	79	113	162	183	235
Washington	22	23	263	30	89	53	79	93	83
West Virginia	119	38	14	35	23	13	38	14	35
Wisconsin	18	33	33	75	136	86	117	146	150
Wyoming	5	10	6	2	1	2	5	6	7
Total	**5,926**	**3,310**	**3,049**	**3,599**	**5,303**	**4,995**	**5,613**	**6,360**	**6,789**

Section III.

Medical Licensing Examinations and Organizations

The United States Medical Licensing Examination™ (USMLE)™

National Board of Medical Examiners
Philadelphia, Pennsylvania

The United States Medical Licensing Examination™ (USMLE™) is a three-step examination for medical licensure in the United States. It is designed to assess a physician's ability to apply knowledge, concepts, and principles, and to demonstrate fundamental patient-centered skills, that are important in health and disease and that constitute the basis of safe and effective patient care. The USMLE is a single examination with three Steps. Each Step is complementary to the others; no Step can stand alone in the assessment of readiness for medical licensure. The USMLE is sponsored by the Federation of State Medical Boards (FSMB) and the National Board of Medical Examiners® (NBME®).

A Composite Committee, appointed by the FSMB and NBME, governs the USMLE. The Composite Committee establishes rules for the USMLE program. Membership includes representatives from the FSMB, NBME, the Educational Commission for Foreign Medical Graduates (ECFMG®), and the American public.

In the United States and its territories, the individual medical licensing authorities ("state medical boards") of the various jurisdictions grant a license to practice medicine. Each medical licensing authority sets its own rules and regulations and requires passing an examination that demonstrates qualification for licensure. Results of the USMLE are reported to these authorities for use in granting the initial license to practice medicine. The USMLE provides them with a common evaluation system for applicants for medical licensure. Because individual medical licensing authorities make their own decisions regarding use of USMLE results, licensure applicants should obtain complete information from the licensing authority. Also, the FSMB can provide general information on medical licensure.

Note: Portions of this chapter reprinted with permission from the *USMLE 2007 Bulletin of Information*, copyright © 2006 by the Federation of State Medical Boards of the United States, Inc, and the National Board of Medical Examiners®; and also from the *2005 NBME Annual Report*, copyright © 2006 by the National Board of Medical Examiners®.

The Three Steps of the USMLE: Step 1, Step 2, and Step 3

Step 1 assesses whether medical school students or graduates can understand and apply important concepts of the sciences basic to the practice of medicine, with special emphasis on principles and mechanisms underlying health, disease, and modes of therapy. Step 1 ensures mastery of not only the sciences that provide a foundation for the safe and competent practice of medicine in the present, but also the scientific principles required for maintenance of competence through lifelong learning.

Step 2 has two separately administered components, the Clinical Knowledge component (Step 2 CK) and the Clinical Skills component (Step 2 CS). The Clinical Skills component became a part of Step 2 in June 2004. Step 2 assesses whether medical school students or graduates can understand and apply the knowledge, skills, and understanding of clinical science considered essential for the provision of patient care under supervision and includes emphasis on health promotion and disease prevention. The inclusion of Step 2 in the USMLE sequence is intended to ensure that due attention is devoted to principles of clinical sciences and basic patient-centered skills that provide the foundation for safe and competent medical practice.

Step 3 assesses whether physicians can apply the medical knowledge and understanding of biomedical and clinical science considered essential for the unsupervised practice of medicine, with emphasis on patient management in ambulatory settings. The inclusion of Step 3 in the USMLE sequence ensures that attention is devoted to the importance of assessing the knowledge of physicians who are assuming independent responsibility for delivering general medical care to patients.

USMLE Eligibility Requirements and Examination Policies

To be eligible to sit for USMLE Step 1, Step 2 CK, and Step 2 CS, an applicant must be in one of the following categories at the time of application and on the examination day:

- A medical student officially enrolled in, or a graduate of, a US or Canadian medical school program leading to the MD degree that is accredited by the Liaison Committee on Medical Education (LCME)
- A medical student officially enrolled in, or a graduate of, a US medical school program leading to the DO degree that is accredited by the American Osteopathic Association (AOA)
- A medical student officially enrolled in, or a graduate of, a medical school outside the United States and Canada and eligible for examination by the ECFMG for its certificate

To be eligible to sit for USMLE Step 3, an applicant must meet all of the following requirements:

- Obtain the MD degree (or its equivalent) or the DO degree
- Obtain a passing performance on Steps 1 and 2 (for those required to take Step 2 CS, both the CS and the CK components of Step 2 will need to be passed in order to be eligible to register for Step 3; see the 2006 USMLE *Bulletin of Information* at www.usmle.org for a detailed description of who is required to take and pass Step 2 CS to be eligible to register for Step 3)
- If a graduate of a medical school outside the United States and Canada, obtain certification by the ECFMG or successfully complete a Fifth Pathway program (see p. 28 for more information)
- Meet the requirements for taking Step 3 set by the medical licensing authority to which the applicant is applying

The USMLE program recommends that for Step 3 eligibility, licensing authorities require the completion, or near completion, of at least 1 training year in a GME program accredited by the Accreditation Council for Graduate Medical Education (ACGME) or the AOA. Applicants should contact the FSMB or the individual licensing authority for complete information on Step 3 eligibility requirements in the state where they plan to be licensed.

Medical students or graduates planning to take USMLE must obtain the most recent information from the appropriate registration entity (see p. 87) before applying for the examination. See the USMLE Web site at www.usmle.org for updated information.

Computer-based Testing

Through Computer-based Testing (CBT), continuous test administration of the USMLE Step 1, Step 2 CK, and Step 3 is available to all examinees. Prometric, a division of Thomson Learning, Inc, provides scheduling and test centers for the USMLE. The Step 1 and Step 2 CK examinations are administered worldwide; the Step 3 examination is administered only in the United States.

Step 2 CS Testing

USMLE Step 2 CS is administered at five regional Clinical Skills Evaluation Centers in the United States:

- Atlanta, Georgia
- Chicago, Illinois
- Houston, Texas
- Philadelphia, Pennsylvania
- Los Angeles, California

Step 2 CS is offered regularly throughout the year at these five sites.

Description of the Examinations

Step 1, Step 2 CK, and Step 3 are administered in sessions of 8 or 9 hours, broken up into sections, or "blocks." The computer keeps track of overall session time, including break time and time allocated for each block of the test. Step 2 CS consists of 12 patient cases. Examinees have 15 minutes for each patient encounter and 10 minutes to record the patient note. The testing session is approximately 8 hours. Further information on examination content and sample test materials for all three steps of the USMLE are available at the USMLE Web site (www.usmle.org).

Step 1

Step 1 has approximately 350 multiple-choice test items, divided into seven 60-minute blocks, administered in one 8-hour testing session. It includes test questions in anatomy, behavioral sciences, biochemistry, microbiology, pathology, pharmacology, and physiology, as well as interdisciplinary topics such as nutrition, genetics, and aging. Step 1 is a broadly based, integrated examination. Test questions commonly require examinees to interpret graphic and tabular material, to identify gross and microscopic pathologic and normal specimens, and to apply basic science knowledge to clinical problems. Step 1 is constructed according to an integrated content outline that organizes basic science material along two dimensions: system and process.

Step 2 CK

Step 2 CK has approximately 370 multiple-choice test items, divided into eight 60-minute blocks, administered in one 9-hour testing session. It includes test questions in internal medicine, obstetrics and gynecology, pediatrics, preventive medicine, psychiatry, surgery, and other areas relevant to provision of care under supervision. The majority of the test questions describe clinical situations and require that examinees provide a diagnosis, prognosis, indication of underlying mechanisms of disease, or the next step in medical care, including preventive measures. Step 2 CK is a broadly based, integrated examination. Interpretation of tables and laboratory data, imaging studies, photographs of gross and microscopic pathologic specimens, and results of other diagnostic studies is frequently required. Step 2 CK is constructed according to an integrated content outline that organizes clinical science material along two dimensions: physician task and disease category.

Step 2 CS

Step 2 CS uses standardized patients, ie, people trained to portray real patients. Examinees are expected to establish rapport with the standardized patients, elicit pertinent historical information from them, perform focused physical examinations, answer questions, and provide counseling when appropriate. After each interaction with a standardized patient, examinees record pertinent history and physical examination findings, list diagnostic impressions, and outline plans for further evaluation, if necessary. The cases cover common and important situations that a physician is likely to encounter in clinics, doctors' offices, emergency departments, and hospital settings in the United States. The sample of cases selected for each examination reflects a balance of cases that is fair and equitable across all examinations. On any examination day, the set of cases will differ from the combination presented the day before or the following day, but each set of cases has a comparable degree of difficulty. The criteria used to create individual examinations focus primarily on presenting complaints and conditions. Presentation categories include, but are not limited to, cardiovascular, constitutional, gastrointestinal, genitourinary, musculoskeletal, neurological, psychiatric, respiratory, and women's health.

Three primary components of Step 2 CS are assessed: (1) data-gathering skills, including history taking and physical examination, and a patient note; (2) communication/interpersonal skills; and (3) spoken English proficiency. Examinees are assessed on their data gathering, physical examination, and communication skills (including spoken English) by the standardized patient, and on their ability to complete the patient note by physician raters.

Examinees must pass all three components in a single administration to obtain the overall designation of passing Step 2 CS. Step 2 CS results are reported as pass or fail, with no numerical scores.

Step 3

Step 3 has approximately 480 multiple-choice test items, divided into blocks of 35 to 50 items, with 45 to 60 minutes to complete each block. In addition, Step 3 has nine computer-based case simulations, with approximately 25 minutes to complete each case. Step 3 is administered in two 8-hour testing sessions.

Step 3 is organized along two principal dimensions: clinical encounter frame and physician task. Step 3 content reflects a data-based model of generalist medical practice in the United States. Encounter frames capture the essential features of circumstances surrounding physicians' clinical activity with patients. They range from encounters with patients seen for the first time for nonemergency problems, to encounters with regular patients seen in the context of continued care, to patient encounters in (life-threatening) emergency situations. Encounters occur in clinics, offices, skilled nursing care facilities, hospitals and emergency departments, and on the telephone.

Step 3 includes Primum® computer-based case simulations (CCS), a test format developed by the NBME that allows the physician taking the test to provide care for a simulated patient. The test-taker decides which diagnostic information to obtain and how to treat and monitor the patient's progress. The computer records each step taken in caring for the patient and scores overall performance. This format permits assessment of clinical decision-making skills in a more realistic and integrated manner than multiple-choice formats.

In the CCS cases, the test-taker may request information from the history and physical examination; order laboratory studies, procedures, and consultants; and start medications and other therapies. Any of the thousands of possible entries that are typed on the "order sheet" are processed and verified by the "clerk." When the test-taker has confirmed that there is nothing further to do, he or she decides when to reevaluate the patient by advancing simulated time. As time passes, the patient's condition changes based on the underlying problem and interventions taken; results of tests are reported and results of interventions must be monitored. The test-taker can suspend the movement of simulated time to consider next steps. While one cannot go back in time, orders can be changed to reflect an updated management plan.

The patient's chart contains, in addition to the order sheet, the reports resulting from orders. By selecting the appropriate chart tabs, the test-taker can review vital signs, progress notes, nurses' notes, and test results. He or she may care for and move the patient among the office, home, emergency department, intensive care unit, and hospital ward.

Preparation for the Examinations

There are no test preparation courses affiliated with or sanctioned by the USMLE program. Information on such courses is not available from the ECFMG, FSMB, NBME, USMLE Secretariat, or medical licensing authorities.

USMLE Steps are broad in scope and are designed to measure the prospective physician's ability to apply knowledge. The best preparation for the USMLE is a general, thorough review of the content reflected in the descriptions for each Step (available at the USMLE Web site).

USMLE Minimum Passing Scores

The USMLE program recommends a minimum passing score for each Step of the USMLE. Minimum passing scores are based on achievement of specified levels of proficiency established prior to administration of examinations. Statistical procedures are employed to ensure that for each Step, the level of proficiency required to pass remains uniform across forms of the examination. As noted in the USMLE *Bulletin of Information* at www.usmle.org, the score required to meet the recommended level of proficiency is reviewed periodically and may be adjusted without prior notice. Notice of adjustments is posted at the USMLE Web site.

In reviewing standards for USMLE examinations, the USMLE Step Committees employ information gathered from a number of sources, including standard-setting surveys. These surveys, which seek opinions on the appropriateness of current USMLE pass/fail standards for each of the Steps, are sent to random samples of examinees, directors of basic and clinical science courses and clinical clerkships, associate deans for academic and student affairs, directors and chief residents from residency programs, members of USMLE test material development committees, executive directors and presidents of all state medical boards, and members of the NBME Board and FSMB Board of Directors.

In addition to surveys, USMLE Step Committees consider the results of content review by standard setting panels. These panels typically consist of physicians who are not otherwise involved in the USMLE program. These panels review the content of the Step examinations and, through a series of exercises, provide data that reflect their opinions on minimally acceptable levels of performance.

Step 1

Details on the performance of examinees taking Step 1 in 2004 and 2005 are provided in Table 26. Data for 2005 are based upon examinees whose results were reported through February 8, 2006. Approximately 16,700 and 16,800 first-time takers from US and Canadian medical schools that grant the MD degree were tested in 2004 and 2005, respectively. First-time takers from non-US/Canadian medical schools numbered approximately 12,300 and 13,500 for the same years. The pass rate for first-time takers from MD-granting US and Canadian medical schools was 93% in 2004 and 94% in 2005.

Table 26
2004-2005 USMLE Step 1 Administrations

	2004		2005*	
	# Tested	% Passing	# Tested	% Passing
Examinees from US/Canadian Schools That Grant:				
MD Degree	18,355	91%	18,290	92%
First-time Takers	16,703	93%	16,799	94%
Repeaters†	1,652	64%	1,491	65%
DO Degree	1,192	69%	1,331	72%
First-time Takers	1,131	70%	1,265	73%
Repeaters†	61	53%	66	53%
Total US/Canadian	*19,547*	*89%*	*19,621*	*90%*
Examinees from Non-US/Canadian Schools				
First-time Takers	12,251	67%	13,488	68%
Repeaters†	5,964	40%	5,911	39%
Total non-US/Canadian	*18,215*	*58%*	*19,399*	*59%*

* Represents data for examinees tested in 2005 and reported through February 8, 2006

† Represents examinations given, not number of different examinees

Because failing examinees generally retake Step 1, the ultimate passing rate across test administrations is expected to increase to approximately 99% for this same group.

Step 2 CK

Details on the performance of examinees taking Step 2 CK in the 2003-2004 and 2004-2005 academic years are provided in Table 27. First-time takers from US and Canadian medical schools granting the MD degree numbered approximately 16,400 for both the 2003-2004 and 2004-2005 periods. First-time takers from non-US/Canadian medical schools numbered approximately 9,900 and 10,400, respectively. The pass rates for first-time takers from MD-granting US and Canadian medical schools was 94% for both periods. As noted with Step 1, given the opportunity for this same group to repeat the examination, the ultimate Step 2 CK passing rate across test administrations is expected to increase to approximately 99%.

Step 2 CS

Details on the performance of examinees taking Step 2 CS in the 2004-2005 academic year (from first day of administration on June 14, 2004 through June 30, 2005) are provided in Table 28. During this period there were approximately 15,800 first-time takers from US and Canadian medical schools that grant the MD degree and 12,700 first-time takers from non-US/Canadian medical schools.

Examinees taking Step 2 CS must pass three separate subcomponents in order to receive an overall pass on Step 2 CS. The three subcomponents are Integrated Clinical Encounter (ICE), Communication and Interpersonal Skills (CIS), and Spoken English Proficiency (SEP). The overall Step 2 CS pass rate for first-time takers from US and Canadian medical schools that grant the MD degree was 96%, and the pass rate for first-time takers from non-US/Canadian medical schools was 83%.

Step 3

Details on the performance of examinees taking Step 3 in 2004 and 2005 are in Table 29. Data for 2005 are based upon examinees whose results were reported through February 8, 2006. First-time takers who were graduates of MD-granting schools in the US and Canada numbered approximately 16,400 in 2004 and 15,900 in 2005. First-time takers who were graduates of non-US/Canadian medical schools numbered approximately 7,700 and 8,300, respectively, for the same years. For 2004 and 2005, the pass rate for first-time takers who were graduates of MD-granting US and Canadian medical schools was 96% for both years. As with Step 1 and Step 2 CK, the ultimate Step 3 passing rate, accounting for repeat attempts, is expected to increase to approximately 99% for this same group.

Table 27
2003-2005 USMLE Step 2 CK Administrations

	2003-2004*		2004-2005*	
	# Tested	% Passing	# Tested	% Passing
Examinees from US/Canadian Schools that Grant:				
MD Degree	17,772	92%	17,803	93%
First-time Takers	16,431	94%	16,447	94%
Repeaters†	1,341	67%	1,356	69%
DO Degree	439	76%	399	85%
First-time Takers	413	80%	386	85%
Repeaters†	26	23%	13	62%
Total US/Canadian	*18,211*	*92%*	*18,202*	*92%*
Examinees from Non-US/Canadian Schools				
First-time Takers	9,862	75%	10,355	77%
Repeaters†	3,178	46%	3,470	50%
Total non-US/Canadian	*13,040*	*68%*	*13,825*	*71%*

* Data for Step 2 CK are provided for examinees tested during the period from July 1 to June 30

†Represents examinations given, not number of different examinees

Table 28
2004-2005 USMLE Step 2 CS Administrations

	2004-2005*	
	# Tested	% Passing
Examinees from US/Canadian Schools that Grant:		
MD Degree	16,124	96%
First-time Takers	15,814	96%
Repeaters†	310	96%
DO Degree	31	87%
First-time Takers	31	87%
Repeaters†	0	NA
Total US/Canadian	*16,155*	*96%*
Examinees from Non-US/Canadian Schools		
First-time Takers	12,708	83%
Repeaters†	973	83%
Total non-US/Canadian	*13,681*	*83%*

* Data for Step 2 CS are provided for examinees tested during the period from June 14, 2004 to June 30, 2005

†Represents examinations given, not number of different examinees

Table 29
2004-2005 USMLE Step 3 Administrations

	2004		2005*	
	# Tested	% Passing	# Tested	% Passing
Examinees from US/Canadian Schools That Grant:				
MD Degree	17,600	94%	16,934	94%
First-time Takers	16,446	96%	15,868	96%
Repeaters†	1,154	69%	1,066	69%
DO Degree	85	93%	58	95%
First-time Takers	81	93%	54	94%
Repeaters†	4	‡	4	‡
Total US/Canadian	17,685	94%	16,992	94%
Examinees from Non-US/Canadian Schools				
First-time Takers	7,668	74%	8,307	75%
Repeaters†	4,791	57%	3,712	52%
Total non-US/Canadian	*12,459*	*68%*	*12,019*	*68%*

* Represents data for examinees tested in 2005 and reported through February 8, 2006

† Represents examinations given, not number of different examinees

‡ Performance data not reported for categories containing fewer than 5 examinees

Communicating About USMLE

Complete information on USMLE is available at the USMLE Web site. Table 30 provides contact information specific to the various Steps. General inquiries regarding the USMLE or inquires for the USMLE Secretariat may be directed to the NBME or the USMLE Secretariat:

USMLE Secretariat
3750 Market St
Philadelphia, PA 19104-3190
215 590-9700
www.usmle.org

Table 30
Contact Information for USMLE

Examination	Type of Applicant	Registration Entity to Contact
Step 1 or Step 2 (CK or CS)	Students and graduates of medical school programs in the US and Canada accredited by the Liaison Committee on Medical Education or students and graduates of medical schools in the US and Canada accredited by the American Osteopathic Association	**NBME** Examinee Support Services, 3750 Market St Philadelphia, PA 19104-3190 215 590-9700 215 590-9457 Fax E-mail: webmail@nbme.org www.nbme.org
Step 1 or Step 2 (CK or CS)	Students and graduates of medical schools outside the US and Canada	**ECFMG** 3624 Market St Philadelphia, PA 19104-2685 215 386-5900 215 386-9196 Fax E-mail: info@ecfmg.org www.ecfmg.org
Step 3	All medical school graduates who have passed Step 1 and Step 2	**FSMB** Department of Examination Services PO Box 619850 Dallas, TX 75261-9850 817 868-4041 817 868-4098 Fax E-mail: usmle@fsmb.org www.fsmb.org – or – **Medical licensing authority**

The Federation of State Medical Boards (FSMB) of the United States, Inc

Founded in 1912, the Federation of State Medical Boards of the United States, Inc (FSMB) is a nonprofit organization composed of the 70 state medical boards of the US and its territories. Through policy development and various initiatives, the FSMB works closely with state medical boards to improve the quality, safety, and integrity of US health care by promoting high standards for physician licensure and practice.

The primary responsibility of each medical licensing board is to protect the public through the regulation of physicians and other health care providers. Within the United States, the organization and activities of each board are determined by state statute, usually referred to as a medical practice act. In general, each state medical board has the authority to license physicians, regulate the practice of medicine, and discipline those who violate the medical practice act.

Physician Data Center

The Federation Physician Data Center is a central repository for formal actions taken against physicians by state licensing and disciplinary boards, the Department of Defense, the US Department of Health and Human Services, and a growing number of international regulatory organizations. The Data Center offers two services used in performing credentialing functions or pre-employment background checks: the *Board Action Data Search* and the *Disciplinary Alert Service*. Both of these services are considered primary source-equivalent by NCQA and JCAHO. The Data Center contains more than 156,000 board actions related to approximately 46,000 physicians dating to the 1960s. This information is available to licensing and disciplinary boards, the military, governmental and private agencies, and organizations involved in the employment and/or credentialing of physicians. The Data Center is also available to the public at www.docinfo.org for a nominal search fee.

Licensure and Assessment Services

In the United States and its territories, a license to practice medicine is a privilege granted only by the individual medical licensing authority of a state or jurisdiction. Each authority sets its own rules and regulations, and each requires successful completion of an examination or certification demonstrating qualification for licensure.

The FSMB, in collaboration with the National Board of Medical Examiners (see p. 92), offers two service packages used by medical licensing authorities for making licensure decisions: The United States Medical Licensing Examination (USMLE™) and the Post-Licensure Assessment System (PLAS).

The USMLE is a 3-step examination taken by individuals preparing for initial medical licensure in the United States. With steps designed to be taken at different times during medical education and training, the USMLE provides a common pathway for evaluating an individual's ability to apply medical knowledge, concepts, and principles to patient care and to demonstrate fundamental patient-centered skills that are important in health and disease and that constitute the basis of safe and effective patient care. (See p. 80 for more information on USMLE.)

The Post-Licensure Assessment System (PLAS), established in 1998, is a joint program of the FSMB and the National Board of Medical Examiners (NBME). The PLAS provides comprehensive services to medical licensing authorities for use in assessing the ongoing clinical competence of licensed physicians. (More information on PLAS is provided on p. 89.)

Federation Credentials Verification Service (FCVS)

The Federation Credentials Verification Service (FCVS) was launched in September 1996 to provide a centralized, uniform process for state medical boards to obtain a verified, primary-source record of physicians' and physician assistants' medical credentials. This service is designed to lighten the workload of credentialing staff and reduce duplication of effort by gathering, verifying, and permanently storing the physician's credentials in a central repository at the FSMB's offices. FCVS obtains primary source verification of medical education, postgraduate training, examination history, board action history, board specialty certification, and identity. This repository of information allows a physician to establish a confidential, lifetime professional portfolio with FCVS which can be forwarded, at the physician's request, to any state medical board that has established an agreement with FCVS as well as other health care entities.

To request an FCVS application, receive more detailed information about the credentialing process, or request a roster of the state medical boards that accept FCVS documents, call toll-free 888 ASK-FCVS (888 275-3287), access the FSMB Web site at www.fsmb.org, or send an e-mail to fcvs@fsmb.org.

Government Relations and Policy

The FSMB monitors federal and state legislation and regulatory policies that affect medical licensure and discipline. Government Services identifies current legislative trends and facilitates communication among member medical boards on issues of mutual interest. Government Services assists state medical boards in legislative and administrative efforts to implement FSMB policy initiatives through formal policy statements, research assistance, written and oral testimony, letters to legislative leadership, etc. The FSMB has played a key role in state and national debates on many prominent issues, including sexual boundaries issues, Internet prescribing, physician profiling, management of chronic pain, oversight of resident physicians, complementary and alternative medicine, and the regulation of office-based surgery.

Publications

The Federation circulates various publications via print and electronic means to inform the public about medical licensing, regulation, discipline, and medical trends. The guidelines and recommendations for handling key issues—such as telemedicine, pain management, physician profiling, and Internet prescribing—are set forth in published policy documents.

On a quarterly basis, the FSMB publishes the *Journal of Medical Licensure and Discipline*, which is distributed to FSMB membership, libraries, medical schools, and subscribers around the world. Member boards and their staffs are served by the monthly newsletter *NewsLine* and the online weekly publication *BoardNet News*. An expansive compendium, the *Exchange*, provides detailed information on physician examination and licensing requirements, along with an overview of medical board structure and disciplinary functions.

The FSMB also publishes all of its policy documents, organizational updates, and the United States Medical Licensing Examination applications, all of which are available online at www.fsmb.org.

Education

The FSMB education department offers various educational programs to its members, including the 3-day Annual Meeting, Board Attorneys Workshop, Executive Management Seminar, and New Executives Orientation. Internet-based workshops for medical board members, senior staff, attorneys, and investigators are also held. CME and CLE credits are available through various program offerings. The FSMB also offers a certification program for state medical board executives and senior staff members based on committee service and participation at FSMB educational events.

Post-Licensure Assessment System (PLAS)

The Post-Licensure Assessment System (PLAS) is a joint program of the FSMB and the National Board of Medical Examiners (NBME®). The PLAS provides a comprehensive inventory of assessment tools that are useful in evaluating the clinical competence of licensed or previously licensed physicians. Such services benefit state medical boards, hospitals, and other organizations interested in assuring that physicians who are providing patient care are competent to do so.

Assessing Medical Knowledge: The Special Purpose Examination (SPEX)

The Special Purpose Examination (SPEX) is a 1-day, multiple-choice examination that tests current knowledge requisite for the general undifferentiated practice of medicine. The examination is intended for physicians who currently hold, or who have previously held, a valid, unrestricted license to practice medicine in a US or Canadian jurisdiction. Licensing boards may require physicians who are applying for licensure by endorsement to successfully complete SPEX if they are some years beyond passage of an initial licensing examination. SPEX is also frequently used to evaluate the cognitive knowledge of physicians seeking licensure reinstatement or reactivation after some period of professional inactivity.

Physicians who hold a current, unrestricted license to practice in a US or Canadian jurisdiction are eligible to apply for the SPEX as a "self-nominated" candidate, independent of any request or approval from a medical licensing board.

The questions used in the SPEX focus on a core of clinical knowledge and relevant underlying basic science principles deemed necessary to form a reasonable foundation for the safe and effective practice of medicine. The examination's content is organized along two primary dimensions: clinical encounter categories (well-care/preventive medicine; acute, circumscribed problems; ill-defined presentations or problems; chronic or progressive illness; emergency conditions; critical care; and behavioral/emotional problems) and physician tasks (data gathering; diagnostic assessment; managing therapy; and applying scientific concepts).

The SPEX has eight blocks of 50 questions; each block lasts approximately 52 minutes. The examination is administered by computer through Prometric Testing Centers, which offers test sites across the United States, its territories, Puerto Rico, the Virgin Islands, and Canada. Test site information is available at www.prometric.com.

SPEX scores are reported directly to the licensing boards for which SPEX is taken and to the examinee. The FSMB maintains a data bank of all SPEX scores to facilitate interstate endorsement. At the request of an examinee, the FSMB will provide certified transcripts of SPEX scores to additional licensing boards.

For more information about the SPEX, call the FSMB Examination Hotline at 817 868-4041 or consult the FSMB Web site at www.fsmb.org.

Multi-modal Clinical Competence Assessment Resources

In addition to SPEX, the PLAS also provides diverse, state-of-the art assessment modalities that, when administered together, generate comprehensive and pertinent data regarding a physician's medical knowledge, clinical judgment, and patient management skills in his or her current or intended area of practice. These tools are utilized by physician evaluation and remediation programs around the country to complement local, performance-based methods of assessment, such as medical record reviews, peer (preceptor) assessment and feedback, patient evaluations, and case-based evaluations of physician care.

Assessment resources currently available through PLAS include Primum® Computer-based Case Simulations (a series of uncued computerized patient simulations); transaction-stimulated recall interviews; standardized, practice-relevant, multiple-choice exams (Internal Medicine, Family Medicine, General Surgery, Obstetrics and Gynecology, Pediatrics, and Psychiatry); and multiple-choice topic module exams (Mechanisms of Disease, Interpreting the Medical Literature, Ethics and Communication, Pharmacotherapeutics with practice-friendly submodules, and Women's Health Care).

Licensing boards, hospitals, group practices, managed care organizations, and other health care organizations will find the in-depth information developed through personalized competence assessments useful in making physician licensure and privileging decisions. Individual physicians may also find assessment services useful in evaluating their clinical competence, particularly if they are at a point of transition in their career or are returning to clinical practice after being away for an extended period of time.

A comprehensive assessment will help determine the strengths and weaknesses a physician has in areas such as practice-relevant medical knowledge, clinical judgment and reasoning, and patient management and communication. Medical organizations may refer a physician for assessment if he or she has been out of practice for an extended period of time or to identify educational activities needed to enhance a physician's practice patterns or to assist in career transitions. Assessments may also be beneficial as part of a review of the clinical capabilities of a physician with personal health concerns, including recovery from disabling illness or injury, neurocognitive concerns, substance abuse, or other issues that may affect practice.

Additional information about the PLAS, its services, and the regional physician evaluation and remediation programs that utilize PLAS assessment resources can be obtained by calling 817 868-4022 or by visiting the FSMB Web site at www.fsmb.org.

Contact Information

Federation of State Medical Boards of the United States, Inc
PO Box 619850
Dallas, TX 75261-9850
817 868-4000
817 868-4099 Fax
www.fsmb.org

National Board of Medical Examiners® (NBME®)

The National Board of Medical Examiners (NBME) is an independent, not-for-profit organization that provides high-quality examinations for the health professions. Protection of the health of the public through state-of-the-art assessment of health professionals is the mission of the NBME, along with a major commitment to research and development in evaluation and measurement. The NBME was founded in 1915 because of the need for a voluntary, nationwide examination that medical licensing authorities could accept as the standard by which to judge candidates for medical licensure. Since that time, it has continued without interruption to provide high-quality examinations for this purpose and has become a model and a resource of international stature in testing methodologies and evaluation in medicine.

Although the NBME's mission is centered on assessment of physicians, it encompasses the spectrum of health professionals along the continuum of education, training, and practice and includes research in evaluation as well as development of assessment instruments.

United States Medical Licensing Examination™ (USMLE™)

The USMLE, cosponsored and co-owned by the NBME and the Federation of State Medical Boards (FSMB), is a three-step examination for medical licensure in the United States. Results of the USMLE are reported to medical licensing authorities in the United States for their use in granting the initial license to practice medicine. The USMLE is the largest NBME examination program. (Information on the USMLE appears on p. 80.)

Services for Medical Schools and Health Professional Organizations

Through a liaison program with medical schools, the NBME fosters communication between the NBME and medical schools, and it provides subject tests in the basic and clinical sciences for the purpose of assessing the educational achievement of individuals in specific subject areas. In 2005, the number of subject examinations administered by medical schools was approximately 151,000. The NBME is augmenting its subject examination program by implementing a system that will allow assembly of customized subject examinations. Customized assessment services will be introduced with a limited number of medical schools in 2006.

The NBME also provides testing, educational, consultative, and research services to a number of medical specialty boards, societies, and health sciences organizations. Services include developing, administering, and analyzing examinations for certification, recertification, in-training, self-assessment, or evaluation of special competence. In 2005, the NBME provided services to 23 organizations, including 50 unique examination programs administered to approximately 65,000 examinees.

In 2003, the NBME introduced a Web-based self-assessment program for basic and clinical science content for US and international medical students and graduates. In 2005, the program added a comprehensive clinical medicine self-assessment. For information on these services, visit the NBME Web site at www.nbme.org.

Services for the International Community

In 2005, the NBME established an International Programs unit. Its goals include to better protect the health of the US and international public, enhance the quality of health care education throughout the world, contribute to the development of state-of-the-art assessment of health professionals internationally, and have an expanded venue for assessment research activities. Services include test item-writing workshops, item sharing, exam development, consultation services, psychometric consultation, editing, and translations. The NBME and the Foundation for Advancement of International Medical Education and Research (FAIMER) of the Educational Commission for Foreign Medical Graduates (ECFMG®) collaborate in international medical education initiatives.

Services for Practicing Physicians

The Post-Licensure Assessment System (PLAS) is a joint activity of the NBME and FSMB and was developed to assist medical licensing authorities in assessing physicians who have already been licensed. The PLAS includes the Special Purpose Examination (SPEX®) and the Assessment Center Program. It provides resources for the comprehensive objective and personalized assessments of physicians for whom there is a question regarding clinical competence, such as endorsement of licensure and licensure reactivation after disciplinary action.

Research and Development

The NBME continually supports intramural research in the fields of clinical skills assessment, advanced methods of testing, and ongoing studies of the validity and reliability of NBME examination programs. In addition, the Edward J. Stemmler Medical Education Research Fund of the NBME supports medical school research relevant to the mission of the NBME.

NBME Certification and Endorsements

The NBME developed and administered its own three-part examination as part of the National Board Certification Program until it was discontinued with the implementation of the USMLE. Certification was awarded to physicians who achieved the following:

- Received the MD degree from an LCME-accredited medical school
- Passed at least one NBME Part or Step examination prior to December 31, 1994 and successfully completed all three Parts/Steps
- Completed, with a satisfactory record, 1 full year (12 months) in a GME program accredited by the Accreditation Council for Graduate Medical Education (accredited internships in Canada were also recognized as meeting this requirement)

Certification by the NBME continues to be used for licensure in the United States for those physicians certified as diplomates prior to implementation of the USMLE and for examinees certified as diplomates who completed a combination of NBME and/or USMLE examinations and passed at least one Part or Step prior to December 31, 1994. The last regular administration of Part I occurred in 1991, Part II in April 1992, and Part III in May 1994. Because some medical students and physicians completed some part of the NBME examination sequence before the implementation of the USMLE, certain combinations of examinations may be considered by medical licensing authorities as comparable to existing examinations. Physicians who passed a combination of examinations should obtain information regarding the acceptability of the combination directly from the medical licensing authority in the jurisdiction where the physician plans to seek licensure.

In 2005, the NBME awarded a total of 63 diplomate certificates, and NBME diplomates requested 8,212 endorsements of certification to medical licensing authorities.

For further information on NBME certification, contact:

NBME
Applicant Services
3750 Market St
Philadelphia, PA 19104
215 590-9700

NBME Web Site

Further information on the NBME and its programs and services is available at www.nbme.org.

National Board of Osteopathic Medical Examiners (NBOME)

Established in 1934, the National Board of Osteopathic Medical Examiners (NBOME) is a not-for-profit corporation dedicated to serving the public and state licensing agencies by administering examinations testing the medical knowledge of those who seek to practice as osteopathic physicians.

The NBOME examinations have been the primary pathway by which osteopathic physicians have applied for licensure to practice osteopathic medicine. A passing score on these examinations verifies a student's adequacy of medical knowledge for practicing osteopathic medicine. Examinations developed by the NBOME are currently accepted in 50 states.

Comprehensive Osteopathic Medical Licensing Examination (COMLEX-USA)

To better assist the state licensing boards in measuring the knowledge required by today's physicians, the NBOME initiated the three-level Comprehensive Osteopathic Medical Licensing Examination (COMLEX-USA) to replace the former three-part NBOME examination series. The COMLEX-USA Level 3 was first administered in February 1995, Level 2 in March 1997, and Level 1 in June 1998.

The COMLEX-USA program is designed to assess the osteopathic medical knowledge considered essential for osteopathic generalist physicians to practice medicine without supervision. COMLEX is constructed in the context of medical problem-solving which involves clinical presentations and physician tasks.

Candidates are expected to utilize the philosophy and principles of osteopathic medicine to solve medical problems. The Clinical Presentation Dimension identifies high-frequency and/or high-impact health issues that osteopathic generalist physicians commonly encounter in practice. The Physician Task Dimension specifies the major steps osteopathic physicians generally undertake in solving medical problems.

Although all three Levels of COMLEX have the same two-dimensional content structure, the depth and emphases of each Level parallel the educational experiences of the candidates. This progressive nature of the COMLEX program ensures the consistency and continuity of the measurement objectives of osteopathic medical licensing examinations.

Level 1

Level 1 emphasizes the medical concepts and principles necessary for understanding the mechanisms of medical problems and disease processes.

Level 1 is a 2-day, written multiple-choice examination covering the basic medical sciences of anatomy, behavioral science, biochemistry, microbiology, osteopathic principles, pathology, pharmacology, physiology, and other relevant areas.

Level 2

Level 2 candidates are expected to demonstrate clinical concepts and principles involved in all steps of medical problem-solving. Level 2 emphasizes the medical concepts and principles necessary for making appropriate medical diagnoses through patient history and physical examination findings.

Level 2 is a 2-day, written multiple-choice examination covering the clinical disciplines of community medicine/ medical humanities, emergency medicine, internal medicine, obstetrics/gynecology, osteopathic principles, pediatrics, psychiatry, surgery, and other areas necessary to solve medical problems.

Level 3

Level 3 candidates are expected to demonstrate clinical concepts and principles necessary for solving medical problems as independently practicing osteopathic generalist physicians. Level 3 emphasizes the medical concepts and principles required to make appropriate patient management decisions.

Level 3 is a 2-day, written multiple-choice examination covering the clinical disciplines of community medicine/medical humanities, emergency medicine, internal medicine, obstetrics/gynecology, osteopathic principles, pediatrics, psychiatry, surgery, and other areas necessary to solve medical problems.

Comprehensive Osteopathic Medical Variable Purpose Examination (COMVEX)

Created by the NBOME, the COMVEX is the newest evaluation instrument offered to osteopathic physicians who need to demonstrate current osteopathic medical knowledge for licensing purposes. It provides the state medical licensing boards a clear evaluation of a candidate's knowledge of current osteopathic medical practices.

The COMVEX is available to candidates through the individual state licensing boards.

Contact Information

National Board of Osteopathic Medical Examiners, Inc
8765 W Higgins Rd, Ste 200
Chicago, IL 60631-4101
773 714-0622
773 714-0631 Fax
www.nbome.org

Section IV.

Information for International Medical Graduates

Educational Commission for Foreign Medical Graduates (ECFMG®)

Stephen S. Seeling, JD
Vice President for Operations
Educational Commission for Foreign Medical Graduates
Philadelphia, Pennsylvania

The Educational Commission for Foreign Medical Graduates (ECFMG®), through its program of certification, assesses the readiness of international medical graduates to enter residency or fellowship programs in the United States that are accredited by the Accreditation Council for Graduate Medical Education (ACGME).

The ECFMG and its organizational members define an international medical graduate (IMG) as a physician who received his/her basic medical degree or qualification from a medical school located outside the United States and Canada. The physician's medical school and graduation year must be listed in the *International Medical Education Directory* (*IMED*) of the Foundation for Advancement of International Medical Education and Research (FAIMER®). The *Directory* contains information supplied by countries about their medical schools. FAIMER is not an accrediting agency. The FAIMER *IMED* is available on the ECFMG Web site at www.ecfmg.org. US citizens who have completed their medical education in schools outside the United States and Canada are considered IMGs; non-US citizens who have graduated from medical schools in the United States and Canada are not considered IMGs.

ECFMG Certification assures directors of ACGME-accredited residency and fellowship programs, and the people of the United States, that IMGs have met minimum standards of eligibility required to enter such programs. ECFMG Certification does not, however, guarantee that such graduates will be accepted into these programs, since the number of applicants often exceeds the number of available positions.

ECFMG Certification is one of the eligibility requirements to take Step 3 of the United States Medical Licensing Examination™ (USMLE™). Medical licensing jurisdictions in the United States also require ECFMG Certification to obtain an unrestricted license to practice medicine.

ECFMG Certification Requirements

Examination Requirements

The examination requirements for ECFMG Certification include passing Step 1 and Step 2 of the USMLE. Step 2 has two separately administered components, the Clinical Knowledge (CK) component and the Clinical Skills (CS) component.

To meet the examination requirements for ECFMG Certification, applicants must satisfy the following requirements:

1. Medical Science Examination Requirement. Step 1 and Step 2 CK of the USMLE are the exams currently administered that satisfy this requirement. To meet the medical science examination requirement for ECFMG Certification, applicants must pass both Step 1 and Step 2 CK within a specified period of time. See *Time Limit for Completing Examination Requirements,* below.

Former Examinations Accepted for ECFMG Certification: The ECFMG also accepts a passing performance on the following former medical science examinations for the purpose of ECFMG Certification: ECFMG Examination, Visa Qualifying Examination (VQE), Foreign Medical Graduate Examination in the Medical Sciences (FMGEMS), and Part I and Part II Examinations of the National Board of Medical Examiners (NBME). Additionally, the ECFMG accepts, for the purpose of its certification, a score of 75 or higher on each of the 3 days of a single administration of the former Federation Licensing Examination (FLEX), if taken prior to June 1985.

Certain combinations of examinations are also acceptable. Applicants who have passed only part of the former VQE, FMGEMS, or the NBME Part I or Part II may combine a passing performance on the basic medical science component of one of these examinations or USMLE Step 1 with a passing performance on the clinical science component of one of the other examinations or USMLE Step 2 CK, provided that the components are passed within the period specified for the examination program.*

2. Clinical Skills Requirement. This requirement includes demonstration of data-gathering and communication skills (including spoken English). Step 2 CS of the USMLE is the exam currently administered that satisfies the clinical skills requirement for ECFMG Certification. Specific time limits for passing Step 2 CS for ECFMG Certification may apply. See *Time Limit for Completing Examination Requirements,* below.

Former Examinations Accepted for ECFMG Certification: Applicants who have **both** passed the former ECFMG Clinical Skills Assessment (CSA®) **and** achieved a score acceptable to ECFMG on an English language proficiency test (such as the Test of English as a Foreign Language™ [TOEFL®] or the former ECFMG English Test) can use these passing performances to satisfy the clinical skills requirement.

Time Limit for Completing Examination Requirements†

ECFMG policy requires that applicants pass those USMLE Steps and Step Components required for ECFMG Certification within a 7-year period. Once an applicant passes a USMLE Step or Step Component, the applicant will have 7 years to pass the other USMLE Step(s) or Step Component(s) required for ECFMG Certification. If an applicant does not pass all required USMLE Steps and Step Components within a maximum of 7 years, the applicant's earliest USMLE passing performance will no longer be valid for ECFMG Certification.

Before implementation of Step 2 CS on June 14, 2004, applicants were required to pass Step 1 and Step 2 CK within a 7-year period for ECFMG Certification. Effective June 14, 2004, applicants must pass Step 1, Step 2 CK, **and Step 2 CS** within a 7-year period for ECFMG Certification; this new 7-year requirement applies to applicants whose earliest USMLE passing performance that is valid for ECFMG Certification is on or after June 14, 2004, as described below.

- **Earliest USMLE Passing Performance Before June 14, 2004**

If an applicant's earliest USMLE passing performance that is valid for ECFMG Certification took place before June 14, 2004, the applicant is required to pass **only Step 1 and Step 2 CK** within a 7-year period for ECFMG Certification. (If the applicant is required to pass Step 2 CS to satisfy the clinical skills requirement for ECFMG Certification, the applicant will not be required to pass Step 2 CS during the same 7-year period in which the applicant must pass Step 1 and Step 2 CK.)

- **Earliest USMLE Passing Performance On or After June 14, 2004**

If an applicant's earliest USMLE passing performance that is valid for ECFMG Certification took place on or after June 14, 2004, the applicant is required to pass Step 1, Step 2 CK, **and Step 2 CS** within a 7-year period for ECFMG Certification.

3. Medical Education Credential Requirements. The physician's medical school and graduation year must be listed in the *International Medical Education Directory* (*IMED*). All IMGs must have had at least 4 credit years (academic years for which credit has been given toward completion of the medical curriculum) in attendance at a medical school listed in *IMED.*

*This policy applies only to ECFMG Certification. Use of the former FLEX Components or the former NBME Parts to fulfill eligibility requirements for Step 3 is no longer accepted. Applicants taking the Steps for the purpose of licensure should refer to *Formerly Administered Examinations* in the USMLE *Bulletin of Information.* Applicants should also contact the medical licensing authority of the jurisdiction where they plan to apply for licensure or the FSMB for specific information on licensure requirements. Additionally, although the ECFMG Examination and FLEX, if taken prior to June 1985, satisfy the medical science examination requirement for ECFMG Certification, they have not been recognized by the US Secretary of Health and Human Services as meeting the medical science examination requirement to obtain a visa to enter the United States (see *Visas*, p. 103).

†This policy applies only to ECFMG Certification. The USMLE program has made specific recommendations to state medical licensing authorities regarding the time to complete all three Steps and the number of attempts allowed to pass each Step or Step component. Refer to *Time Limit and Number of Attempts Allowed to Complete All Steps*, *Retakes*, and *Official Performance of Record for Examinees Retaking a Previously Passed Step* in the USMLE *Bulletin of Information.* Applicants should also contact the medical licensing authority of the jurisdiction where they plan to apply for licensure or the FSMB, since licensure requirements vary among jurisdictions.

Applicants for ECFMG Certification must document the completion of all requirements for, and receipt of, the final medical diploma. ECFMG verifies every applicant's medical school diploma with the appropriate officials of the medical school that issued the diploma. When ECFMG sends the applicant's medical diploma to the medical school for verification, ECFMG will request the medical school to include the applicant's final medical school transcript when the school returns the verification of the medical diploma to ECFMG. An applicant's credentials are not considered complete until ECFMG receives verification of the medical diploma and final medical school transcript directly from the medical school.

Standard ECFMG Certificate

The ECFMG issues the Standard ECFMG Certificate to applicants who meet all of the examination and medical education credential requirements. Applicants must also pay any outstanding charges on their ECFMG financial accounts before their certificates are issued. Standard ECFMG Certificates are sent approximately 2 weeks after all of these requirements have been met.

A Standard ECFMG Certificate includes:

- The name of the applicant
- The applicant's USMLE/ECFMG Identification Number
- The dates that examination requirements were met
- The date that the certificate was issued
- **If applicable**, the date(s) through which the passing performance on certain exam(s) remain valid for the purpose of entry into graduate medical education (GME). (See *Validity of Examinations for Entry into GME*, below.)

The Standard ECFMG Certificate may be used for entry into accredited GME programs in the United States.

Validity of Examinations for Entry into GME

Clinical Skills Examinations

For applicants who satisfy the clinical skills requirement by passing Step 2 CS, this passing performance is not subject to expiration for the purpose of entering GME programs.

For applicants who satisfied the clinical skills requirement for ECFMG Certification by passing the former ECFMG CSA and an English language proficiency test, passing performance on the CSA may be subject to expiration for the purpose of entering GME programs, as described below.

- Passing performances on **CSA administrations that took place on or after June 14, 2001**, are not subject to expiration for the purpose of entering GME programs. Applicants who are certified by ECFMG and whose Standard ECFMG Certificate lists a "valid through" date for an administration of the CSA that took place on or after June 14, 2001, may request a permanent validation sticker online by accessing OASIS or by completing a *Special Request for Permanent Validation Sticker* (Form 295) and submitting it to ECFMG. Applicants can access OASIS and Form 295 on the ECFMG Web site.

- Passing performances on **CSA administrations that took place before June 14, 2001**, are valid for 3 years from the date passed for the purpose of entering GME programs. The date through which passing performance on the CSA remains valid for entry into GME (the CSA "valid through" date) will be listed on the applicant's Standard ECFMG Certificate. If the applicant has entered a program before expiration of the valid through date, the applicant may request permanent validation. This means that the CSA date is no longer subject to expiration. To request permanent validation, the applicant and an authorized official of the training institution must complete a *Request for Permanent Validation* (Form 246). On receipt of such official documentation, ECFMG will provide a "permanent validation" sticker to be affixed to the certificate. If an applicant who passed CSA before June 14, 2001, does not enter a GME program within 3 years of the CSA pass date, the applicant's CSA passing performance will expire for the purpose of entering GME. Before entering a program, these applicants must pass Step 2 CS. Passing performance on Step 2 CS does not expire for the purpose of entry into GME.

English Examinations

Passing performances on the English language proficiency test (such as the TOEFL exam or the former ECFMG English Test) are not subject to expiration for the purpose of entering GME programs, regardless of the date passed. Applicants who are certified by ECFMG and whose Standard ECFMG Certificate lists a "valid through" date for an English language proficiency test may request a permanent validation sticker online by accessing OASIS or by completing a *Special Request for Permanent Validation*

Table 31
Examinee Performance for International Medical Graduates/Students Taking USMLE Step 1 and Step 2 (CK and CS) Examinations

	USMLE Step 1 January 1, 2005 - December 31, 2005			USMLE Step 2 CK July 1, 2004 - June 30, 2005			USMLE Step 2 CS June 14, 2004 - June 30, 2005		
	Number of Administrations	Number Passing	Percent Passing	Number of Administrations	Number Passing	Percent Passing	Number of Administrations	Number Passing	Percent Passing
Total	**19,362**	**11,450**	**59**	**13,832**	**9,750**	**70**	**13,478**	**11,200**	**83**
First-time Takers	13,445	9,164	68	10,357	8,001	77	11,473	9,612	84
Repeaters	5,917	2,286	39	3,475	1,749	50	2,005	1,588	79
US Citizens	**5,009**	**2,285**	**46**	**3,085**	**1,807**	**59**	**2,397**	**2,113**	**88**
First-time Takers	2,786	1,563	56	1,980	1,308	66	2,123	1,883	89
Repeaters	2,223	722	32	1,105	499	45	274	230	84
Foreign Citizens	**14,353**	**9,165**	**64**	**10,747**	**7,943**	**74**	**11,081**	**9,087**	**82**
First-time Takers	10,659	7,601	71	8,377	6,693	80	9,350	7,729	83
Repeaters	3,694	1,564	42	2,370	1,250	53	1,731	1,358	78

Notes: Step 1 first-time takers are those examinees with no prior Step 1 and no prior NBME Part I examinations.
Step 2 CK first-time takers are those examinees with no prior Step 2 CK and no prior NBME Part II examinations.
Step 2 CS first-time takers are those examinees with no prior Step 2 CS and no prior ECFMG CSA examinations.
Administrations include those with results of Pass, Fail, Incomplete, Indeterminate, and Withheld.
The data for repeaters represents examinations given, not examinees.
Citizenship is as of the time of entrance into medical school.
Source: ECFMG Examination History. Data current as of February 9, 2006.

Sticker (Form 295) and submitting it to ECFMG. Applicants can access OASIS and Form 295 on the ECFMG Web site.

Important Note: The preceding discussion of validity and expiration of examinations, and the "valid through" and "valid indefinitely" designations on the Standard ECFMG Certificate (if applicable), are relevant **only** for the purpose of entry into US GME programs. They do **not** pertain to eligibility for USMLE Step 3 or to any time limits imposed by medical licensing authorities or other entities for the completion of all USMLE Steps.

Step 1 and Step 2 of the USMLE

The USMLE is a single, three-step examination for medical licensure in the United States that provides a common system to evaluate applicants for medical licensure. The USMLE is sponsored by the Federation of State Medical Boards of the United States, Inc (FSMB) and the NBME. The USMLE is governed by a committee consisting of members of the FSMB, NBME, ECFMG, and the American public. The USMLE Steps 1, 2, and 3 replaced FLEX and the NBME Parts I, II, and III.

The ECFMG determines whether international medical students/graduates are eligible to take USMLE Step 1 and Step 2 and registers eligible applicants to take these exams for the purpose of ECFMG Certification. The NBME registers eligible students/graduates of US and Canadian medical schools/programs accredited by the Liaison Committee on Medical Education or the American Osteopathic Association to take Step 1 and Step 2.

USMLE Step 1 and Step 2 CK are multiple-choice examinations that are administered by computer. Prometric, a division of Thomson Learning, Inc, provides scheduling and test centers for Step 1 and Step 2 CK. These exams are delivered throughout the year at Prometric Test Centers worldwide.

Step 2 CS uses standardized patients in simulated clinical encounters to evaluate clinical and communication skills. Step 2 CS is administered at clinical skills evaluation centers in Atlanta, Chicago, Houston, Los Angeles, and Philadelphia in the United States.

Table 31 shows the performance of IMGs for recent administrations of Step 1 and Step 2 (CK and CS).

Standard ECFMG Certificates Issued in 2005

During 2005, 11,535* Standard ECFMG Certificates were issued. Table 32 shows the distribution of recipients of Standard ECFMG Certificates by country of medical school and citizenship. In 2005, medical schools in India and Pakistan had the largest number of recipients: 2,790 (24.2%) were graduates of Indian medical schools and 682 (5.9%) of the recipients received their medical degrees in Pakistan.

Based upon country of citizenship, citizens of India formed the largest group of recipients. Of the certificates issued in 2005, 2,744 (23.8%) were to Indian citizens. Citizens of the United States were the second largest group with 1,932 (16.7%) recipients.

Table 32
Standard ECFMG Certificates Issued in 2005: Distribution of Recipients by Country of Medical School and Citizenship

Country	Country of Medical School		Country of Citizenship	
	Number	%	Number	%
Argentina	123	1.1	107	0.9
Australia	113	1.0	70	0.6
Bangladesh	111	1.0	97	0.8
Brazil	109	0.9	109	0.9
Bulgaria	56	0.5	47	0.4
Canada	0	0.0	205	1.8
Cayman Islands	76	0.7	0	<0.1
China	443	3.8	444	3.8
Colombia	227	2.0	217	1.9
Cuba	133	1.2	132	1.1
Dominica	472	4.1	5	0.0
Dominican Republic	190	1.6	80	0.7
Egypt	185	1.6	173	1.5
Ethiopia	49	0.4	56	0.5
Germany	191	1.7	157	1.4
Ghana	71	0.6	85	0.7
Grenada	439	3.8	5	<0.1
Hungary	59	0.5	14	0.1
India	2,790	24.2	2,744	23.8
Iran	252	2.2	273	2.4
Ireland	171	1.5	78	0.7
Israel	177	1.5	74	0.6
Japan	83	0.7	81	0.7
Jordan	125	1.1	141	1.2
Lebanon	152	1.3	159	1.4
Mexico	174	1.5	107	0.9
Myanmar	72	0.6	74	0.6
Nepal	106	0.9	133	1.2
Netherlands Antilles	345	3.0	0	0.0
Nigeria	286	2.5	294	2.5
Pakistan	682	5.9	620	5.4
Peru	104	0.9	109	0.9
Philippines	436	3.8	358	3.1
Poland	150	1.3	73	0.6
Romania	168	1.5	153	1.3
Russia	189	1.6	125	1.1
South Korea	127	1.1	119	1.0
Syria	174	1.5	166	1.4
Thailand	84	0.7	81	0.7
Turkey	84	0.7	77	0.7
Ukraine	110	1.0	69	0.6
United Kingdom	100	0.9	117	1.0
USA	0	0.0	1,932	16.7
USSR	0	0.0	65	0.6
Venezuela	95	0.8	95	0.8
Countries with fewer than 50 recipients	1,252	10.9	1,215	10.5
Totals	**11,535**	**100**	**11,535**	**100**

Notes: Citizenship is as of the time of entrance into medical school.

For country of medical school, the countries of the former USSR are represented separately.

Percentages may not equal 100% due to rounding.

*The availability of exam results for some examinees taking Step 2 CS during the initial months of test administration in 2004 was delayed until early 2005. As a result, the number of certificates issued in 2005 is higher than it would have been, had this delay not occurred.

Electronic Residency Application Service (ERAS®)

The Association of American Medical Colleges (AAMC) developed the Electronic Residency Application Service (ERAS), to transmit residency applications, letters of recommendation, Medical Student Performance Evaluations (MSPEs), transcripts, and other supporting documents to residency program directors via the Internet. ERAS is available to IMGs through ECFMG, the designated Dean's Office for all IMGs.

Most medical specialties participate in ERAS. Programs in participating specialties require applicants to apply for positions using ERAS.

For a list of specialties participating in ERAS in 2007, visit http://services.aamc.org/eras/erasstats/par/.

Additional specialties may use ERAS for residency programs beginning in July 2008. Applicants should contact residency program directors for specific requirements and deadlines.

For information or to apply, visit the ECFMG Web site at www.ecfmg.org/eras. Applicants may also contact:

ERAS
ECFMG
3624 Market St
Philadelphia, PA 19104-2685
E-mail: eras-support@ecfmg.org
215 386-5900
215 222-5641 Fax

Visas

To obtain a visa to enter the United States to perform services as members of the medical profession or to receive GME, certain foreign national physicians are required, under the provisions of Public Law 94-484, to pass NBME Part I and Part II examinations or an examination determined to be equivalent for this purpose. The Secretary of Health and Human Services has recognized USMLE Step 1 and Step 2 as well as the former Visa Qualifying Examination (VQE) and the Foreign Medical Graduate Examination in the Medical Sciences (FMGEMS) as equivalent to NBME Part I and Part II examinations for the purposes of PL 94-484. To obtain additional information on visa requirements, foreign national physicians should refer to the following Web sites:

- ECFMG Exchange Visitor Sponsorship Program
  www.ecfmg.org/evsp
- US Embassies or Consulates of the US Department of State (DOS)
  www.state.gov
- Immigration Bureaus of the US Department of Homeland Security (DHS)
  www.dhs.gov

Exchange Visitor Sponsorship Program

The ECFMG is authorized by the United States Department of State (DOS) to sponsor foreign national physicians as J-1 Exchange Visitors in GME or training programs. The objectives of this program are to enhance international exchange in the field of medicine and to promote mutual understanding between the people of the United States and other countries through the interchange of persons, knowledge, and skills.

The program is administered by ECFMG in accordance with the provisions set forth in an agreement between the ECFMG and the DOS and the federal regulations established to implement the Mutual Educational and Cultural Exchange Act. The ECFMG is responsible for ensuring that all Exchange Visitor Physicians and host institutions comply with the federal requirements for participation. The ECFMG issues a Certificate of Eligibility for Exchange Visitor J-1 Status (Form DS-2019) for qualified applicants. This document must be processed through the United States Embassy or Consulate of the US DOS and/or the immigration bureaus of the US DHS.

The Federal regulations refer to Exchange Visitor Physicians seeking J-1 sponsorship in clinical programs as *alien physicians.* These applicants must meet, among other requirements, a number of general requirements, which are detailed in the ECFMG's application materials for J-1 visa sponsorship. At a minimum, applicants must:

- Pass USMLE Step 1 and Step 2 CK (and/or an acceptable combination of the former FMGEMS, NBME, or VQE examinations) (*Note:* The former 1-day ECFMG Examination and FLEX do not meet the requirements for J-1 visa sponsorship.)

Table 33
Exchange Visitor Sponsorship Program for Physicians: Number of J-1 Physicians in Graduate Medical Education or Training Programs in the United States, July 1, 2004, to June 30, 2005

Specialty	Count
Allergy and Immunology	8
Anesthesiology	170
Colon and Rectal Surgery	9
Dermatology	13
Emergency Medicine	31
Family Medicine	348
General Preventive Med, Occupational Med, Aerospace Med, & Public Health	7
Internal Medicine	2,850
Internal Medicine/Family Practice	1
Internal Medicine/Pediatrics	34
Internal Medicine/Preventive Medicine	1
Internal Medicine/Psychiatry	8
Medical Education	11
Medical Genetics	16
Molecular Genetic Pathology	3
Neurological Surgery	47
Neurology	222
Nuclear Medicine	8
Obstetrics and Gynecology	153
Ophthalmology	54
Orthopedic Surgery	60
Otolaryngology	19
Pathology	69
Pathology - Anatomic and Clinical	177
Pediatrics	707
Pediatrics/Medical Genetics	1
Physical Medicine and Rehabilitation	24
Plastic Surgery	15
Preventive Medicine	1
Psychiatry	382
Psychiatry/Neurology	1
Radiation Oncology	8
Radiology	1
Radiology - Diagnostic	136
Surgery - General	452
Thoracic Surgery	58
Transitional Year	12
Urology	33
Total	**6,150**

- Hold a Standard ECFMG Certificate without expired examination dates, if applicable. *Note:* See *Validity of Examinations for Entry into GME*, above, for important information (Graduates of LCME- and AOA-accredited US and Canadian medical schools/programs are not required to be ECFMG-certified.)
- Hold a contract or an official letter of offer for a position in a GME or training program that is affiliated with a medical school
- Provide a statement of need from the Ministry of Health of the country of most recent legal permanent residence. This statement must provide written assurance that the country needs specialists in the area in which the Exchange Visitor will receive training and that he/she will return to the country upon completion. (*Note:* If permanent residence is in a country other than that of citizenship, the Ministry of Health letter must come from the country of most recent legal permanent residence.)

The duration of stay for a J-1 Exchange Visitor Physician is limited to the time typically required to complete the advanced medical education program. This refers to the specialty and subspecialty certification requirements published by the American Board of Medical Specialties (ABMS®). Participation is further limited to 7 years and is reserved for those progressing in approved training programs.

J-1 Exchange Visitor Physicians sponsored for participation in nonclinical programs primarily involved with observation, consultation, teaching, or research are categorized as *research scholars*. Unlike alien physicians, participants in these programs generally do not have to pass US medical licensing or English examinations and are not required to be ECFMG-certified. Research scholars are limited to activities involving no patient contact or only incidental patient contact. The maximum period of participation for research scholars is 3 years.

Table 33 shows that the ECFMG sponsored 6,150 Exchange Visitor Physicians in US GME or training programs for the academic year July 1, 2004, to June 30, 2005. In the alien physician category, the ECFMG sponsored 3,925 in clinical residency (specialty) programs and 2,169 in clinical fellowships (subspecialty training) in 2004-2005. A total of 56 foreign nationals were sponsored in the research scholar category. Foreign nationals from India and Pakistan represented approximately one quarter of ECFMG-sponsored J-1 physicians for this period.

For application materials and specific information on ECFMG sponsorship, applicants should visit the ECFMG Web site at www.ecfmg.org/evsp. Applicants may also contact:

Educational Commission for Foreign Medical Graduates
Exchange Visitor Sponsorship Program
3624 Market St
Philadelphia, PA 19104-2685
215 823-2121
215 386-9766 Fax

Certification Verification Service (CVS)

The ECFMG's Certification Verification Service provides primary source confirmation of the ECFMG certification status of IMGs. The Joint Commission on Accreditation of Healthcare Organizations (JCAHO) has determined that an accredited health organization will satisfy the JCAHO requirement for primary source verification of medical school completion for IMGs if it confirms directly with the ECFMG that an applicant possesses a valid Standard ECFMG Certificate.

The ECFMG will confirm an applicant's certification status when a request is received from a medical licensing authority, residency program director, hospital, or other organization that, in the judgment of ECFMG, has a legitimate interest in such information. For status reports sent to medical licensing authorities, the request can also be sent to ECFMG by the applicant. Requesting organizations must normally secure and retain the applicant's signed authorization to obtain certification information. Please note that there may be a fee for this service.

Requests for confirmation must contain the applicant's name, date of birth, and USMLE/ECFMG Identification Number, as well as the name and address of the organization to which the confirmation should be sent. Confirmations are mailed to the requesting organization within approximately 2 weeks. Confirmations are not sent to applicants directly.

For individuals who apply to residency programs through ERAS, the ECFMG automatically sends an electronic ECFMG status report, at the time that their applications are processed, to all of the programs to which they applied. If an applicant's ECFMG certification status changes during the ERAS application process, the ECFMG will automatically send an updated status report to all programs to which the applicant applied.

To obtain information, request form(s), or make an online request, refer to the CVS home page on the ECFMG Web site at www.ecfmg.org/cvs or contact:

Educational Commission for Foreign Medical Graduates
CVS Department
PO Box 13679
Philadelphia PA 19101-3679
215 386-5900

Contact Information

Interested individuals can access the ECFMG *Information Booklet* and apply online for USMLE Step 1 and Step 2 by visiting the ECFMG Web site at www.ecfmg.org. The ECFMG Web site also provides access to important updates, ECFMG's online services, and more than 50 ECFMG publications and forms.

Individuals who do not have access to the Internet may contact the ECFMG for assistance.

ECFMG
3624 Market St
Philadelphia, PA 19104-2685
215 386-5900
215 386-9196 Fax
E-mail: info@ecfmg.org
www.ecfmg.org

Immigration Overview for International Medical Graduates

Robert D. Aronson, partner
Ingber & Aronson, Minneapolis, Minnesota

This article outlines current immigration laws and policies that affect the physician community. While the September 11 attacks have had a major impact on immigration policy and attitudes—including the entire restructuring of the immigration function into the Department of Homeland Security—there are two salient points of note: first, that as a nation of laws, we continue to have in place predictable and workable immigration provisions which enable deserving foreign nationals to enter this country consistent with our national traditions; and second, given the emerging shortage of physicians in the workforce and the misdistribution patterns largely affecting rural and inner city communities, there have been a number of new initiatives of particular relevance to the immigration of international medical graduates (IMGs).

This article deals with three broad areas of relevance to the immigration of IMGs:

1. Temporary, nonimmigrant visa options for foreign physicians
2. The J-1 waiver process for physicians
3. Options in order to qualify for permanent residence

Immigration Law Overview

All foreign nationals enter the United States in one of two broad immigration categories—either under a temporary, nonimmigrant visa or as a permanent resident. There are comparative advantages to both these categories. In the case of the temporary, nonimmigrant visa classifications, it is usually possible to gain this type of immigration coverage in a relatively short time. The two most commonly used temporary, nonimmigrant classifications by IMGs are the J-1 Exchange Visitor program and the H-1B Temporary Worker classification. Both these classifications, however, limit a physician's duration of residence in the United States and impose strict limitations on the range of employment authorization, although they do have the advantage of being relatively quick to obtain. In contrast, permanent residence provides a foreign national with both an unlimited duration of residence and full, unrestricted employment authorization, although the processing time is much greater.

Temporary, Nonimmigrant Classifications

Most IMGs in graduate medical education (GME) programs arrive under the J-1 Exchange Visitor program, although the H-1B Temporary Worker category is becoming increasingly utilized.

The J-1 program is administered by the US Department of State and is intended to provide a broad range of foreign nationals with educational, employment, and training opportunities in the United States. To apply for a J-1 visa, an IMG must first obtain certification from the Educational Commission for Foreign Medical Graduates (ECFMG), which is the implementing agency for the J-1 Exchange Visitor program for physicians. To gain an ECFMG Certificate, an IMG needs to fulfill the following requirements:

1. Pass stipulated examinations—currently, the US Medical Licensing Examination (USMLE), Steps 1 and 2 Clinical Knowledge and Clinical Skills—to establish medical competence and English language competence
2. Pass the ECFMG English language examination to establish English language competence
3. Possess an MD degree from a foreign medical school listed in the *International Medical Education Directory* of the Foundation for Advancement of International Medical Education and Research (FAIMER®)

All J-1 trainees must receive ECFMG certification, except for graduates of Canadian medical schools, who are exempt from this requirement because Canadian medical education and training are accredited under US standards (or considered equivalent to US education/training).

Upon entry to the United States, an IMG is authorized to pursue a clinical GME program for up to 7 years to achieve stipulated training objectives. Each year, the GME program, in conjunction with the IMG, needs to file an extension application with the ECFMG.

Without exception, all J-1 physicians engaged in clinical training activities are subject to a mandatory 2-year home residence obligation, regardless of country of citizenship or last permanent residence. *Note:* This 2-year home residence requirement applies to every physician who enters the United States under an ECFMG-sponsored J-1 clinical training program. To ultimately qualify for permanent residence and/or an H-1B visa, an IMG must either return to his/her home country for a 2-year period or obtain a waiver of this 2-year obligation.

J-1 Waiver Strategies

As noted above, all ECFMG-sponsored J-1 physicians—regardless of country of citizenship—are subject to an obligation to return to their home country for a mandatory 2-year period of time. Unless and until this 2-year home residence is either fulfilled (ie, by returning specifically to the home country) or waived (ie, eliminated), a physician under law is barred from obtaining an H-1B visa and/or permanent resident status. Therefore, it is critically important for long-term immigration prospects for a J-1 physician to obtain a waiver of the 2-year home residence requirement. US laws do contain various provisions enabling J-1 physicians to obtain such waivers.

A waiver of this obligation is available only on the basis of at least one the following three grounds:

- If the J-1 physician will suffer from persecution in his/her home country or country of last permanent residence
- If fulfillment of the obligation will subject a US citizen spouse or child to exceptional hardship
- Based upon a recommendation issued by a government agency interested in the physician's continued residence/employment in the United States

Without question, the vast majority of J-1 physicians who receive waivers do so through recommendations issued by government agencies. Generally speaking, such waivers fall within the following three basic patterns:

- Employment by a federal agency, such as the Department of Veterans Affairs
- Recognition of outstanding academic and research achievements, as determined by the Department of Health and Human Services
- Service to medically underserved patient populations, so as to allow either a state department of health or a federal agency to recommend a waiver as a matter of public interest

Statistically, the vast majority of J-1 physicians have obtained waivers through a program known as the Conrad State 30 program, which essentially empowers each state to recommend waivers for up to 30 physicians per fiscal year. These waivers specifically require the physician to practice medicine (either primary care or specialty) in a designated medically underserved location. Effective December 2004, five waivers can be issued if the physician's practice benefits the indigent and the medically underserved, even if the physician's actual practice site is not in a designated medically underserved area. Furthermore, the physician needs to practice medicine in the community for at least 3 years, working specifically in H-1B status. Any premature departure from the community could result in a loss of the waiver as well as immigration status.

The majority of waivers are issued by the departments of health of the various states. Most states now recommend waivers to medical specialists as well as to primary care practitioners. In addition, various federal agencies also maintain J-1 waiver programs, including the Department of Health and Human Services, the Delta Regional Commission, and the Appalachian Regional Commission. Most federal agencies, however, limit their waiver programs to primary care physicians, even though the law was liberalized in December 2004 to cover medical specialists. The federal agencies do not, though, have any quota limitation on the number of waivers that they can recommend.

H1-B Temporary Worker

Instead of taking part in the J-1 Exchange Visitor program, with its home residence obligation, an increasing number of foreign physicians are entering the United States under the H-1B Temporary Worker provisions. This visa classification enables a foreign national to enter the United States for professional-level employment for up to 6 years. In most instances, H-1B coverage can be obtained within approximately 60-90 days, although there are provisions for expediting the processing of an immigration case. The H-1B quota of 65,000 is normally exhausted early on in the federal fiscal year. Many physicians who obtain J-1 waivers, however, are exempted from the H-1B quota.

To qualify for H-1B benefits, an IMG must meet the following four criteria:

- Possession of a full, unrestricted state medical license or the "appropriate authorization" for the position
- An MD degree or a full, unrestricted foreign license
- English language competence as established either through graduation from an accredited medical school or by holding an ECFMG Certificate
- Passage of the Federation Licensing Examination (FLEX) or its equivalents—the National Board of Medical Examiners (NBME), Parts I, II, and III, or the USMLE, Steps 1, 2, and 3

As a result of the FLEX equivalency issue, most Canadian physicians do not qualify for H-1B benefits. The standard Canadian medical credential—the Licentiate of the Medical Council of Canada (LMCC)—is widely accepted among the states for medical licensure purposes. Therefore, most Canadian physicians have traditionally not had any reason to sit for the FLEX or its equivalents. In this manner, H-1B immigration requirements have established different credentialing standards from those of the state medical licensing boards, which have traditionally been the primary judge of physician competence.

Permanent Residence Strategies

A foreign national can qualify for permanent residence in various ways, ranging from familial relationships with US citizens or permanent residents to fear of persecution that would merit refugee entitlement. In most instances, though, an IMG will need to qualify for permanent residence based upon an employment position. There are three basic pathways to permanent residence based upon employment as a physician.

Pathway One

The "normal" route to permanent residence involves a three-step process. The first and arguably most complex stage is the Labor Certification Application process. This is a procedure conducted under the auspices of the US Department of Labor to establish that the employment of a foreign national will in no manner harm the US labor market, particularly by taking a job away from a fully qualified US worker. Therefore, acting under a complex recruitment/advertisement procedure, the employer needs to show that the IMG is not simply the best-qualified applicant for the position but is the only fully qualified candidate for the specific position. Effective March 28, 2005, the Labor Certification Application process was reengineered into the PERM Program, which places certain constraints on this process but speeds up considerably the processing time for such applications.

After completing the Labor Certification Application process, the employer needs to submit an Immigrant Visa Petition to the US Citizenship and Immigration Services (CIS, formerly the Immigration and Naturalization Service), establishing the complete suitability of the IMG for the position. Upon approval of this petition, the IMG is then able to actually apply for permanent residence either through a CIS District Office (adjustment of status) or through a US Consular post (consular processing).

Note: An IMG must possess either an ECFMG Certificate or an MD degree from an accredited medical school (ie, generally US or Canadian). Also, an IMG cannot finalize the application for permanent residence status if he/she has an unfulfilled or unwaived J-1 2-year home residence obligation.

Pathway Two

A second pathway to employment-related permanent residence is based upon National Interest Waiver criteria. In this instance, an IMG has a streamlined, expedited pathway to permanent residence if it can be shown that the IMG's employment as a physician carries potential major benefits to areas of high national interest. Under current law, primary care physicians working in designated medically underserved areas can qualify for permanent residence pursuant to a National Interest Waiver. Any physician using this pathway, however, has an obligation of working in a designated medically underserved community for a minimum of 5 years. Furthermore, National Interest Waiver eligibility is limited to primary care physicians (unless the physician is working in a VA facility, in which case medical specialists can also obtain permanent residence through this procedure).

Pathway Three

A third option to permanent residence is available to physicians of extraordinarily high professional capabilities, working either in clinical practice or in academic medicine. Such individuals may qualify for permanent residence under an expedited procedure established for Aliens of Extraordinary Ability and Outstanding Professors or Researchers.

New Legal Developments

The state-based waiver program is now up for extension by Congress. Two years ago, the waiver program was enlarged and extended, and it is anticipated that it may be extended on a permanent basis. This program has become a popular and frequently used initiative within the states that give state health care planners expanded flexibility to address a state's need for expanded physician coverage.

The entire immigration function has been shifted from the Immigration and Naturalization Service to an entirely new federal agency, US Citizenship and Immigration Services (CIS), which is part of the Department of Homeland Security. This restructuring reflects a new focus on security-related reviews of immigration requests. While there have been some delays, immigration requests continue to be adjudicated and approved and visas granted, as required by the law.

Many IMGs, particularly from third world countries, have traditionally applied for their visas through US Consulates in the neighboring countries of Canada or Mexico. A new law creates major new restrictions on visa processing in these countries, although some concessions have been granted to physicians who intend to work in designated medically underserved communities.

The H-1B quota has been reduced to 65,000, which is grossly insufficient to serve the needs of US employers seeking the services of H-1B professionals. Accordingly, these numbers recurrently run out in the early part of the fiscal year, meaning that foreign nationals whose H-1B petitions are filed after visa numbers are exhausted face long waits until the H-1B numbers again become available in the next federal fiscal year. Congress is currently considering reform legislation to enlarge the number of H-1B visas.

A new law has created major new bars to permanent residence for foreign nationals who have resided illegally within the United States for extended periods of time. This provision is certainly not targeted directly at physicians but is rather an across-the-board provision intended to create a major new disincentive for violating US immigration laws.

Certainly, the events of 9/11 have affected immigration prospects for physicians as well. Under present standards, foreign nationals from selected countries in the Middle East are subject to enhanced security and background screening requirements. They are also greatly restricted in processing for visas through US Consulates located in third countries. Furthermore, any lapse in immigration status or violations of employment eligibility could present major future problems for qualifying for future immigration benefits.

But when all is said and done, we as a nation have complex and ever expanding needs for physicians, particularly those willing to serve in isolated areas and those willing to treat minorities, ethnic populations, and the indigent. Over the years, foreign physicians have been one of the most effective physician population groups for addressing medically underserved populations, and our immigration laws have developed several meaningful and effective initiatives intended to facilitate the relocation of foreign physicians into positions of maximum benefit to various US population groups.

Robert D. Aronson is the managing partner for Ingber & Aronson, a law firm that practices exclusively in the area of immigration and nationality law. The major area of his practice deals with immigration matters for foreign physicians and US medical institutions nationwide. He received his law degree from Indiana University and was a Fulbright Fellow at Harvard Law School and Moscow State University (Russia). Mr. Aronson has held various leadership positions on immigration matters for international physicians within the medical, legal, academic, and governmental communities.

Section V.

Federal and National Programs and Activities

Licensure in the US Armed Forces

Department of the Air Force

Joseph J. Legan, Lt Col, USAF, MC, SFS
Chief, Clinical Quality Management Division

Kimberly G. Coltman, Lt Col, USAF, NC
Chief, Credentialing and Privileging Policy
Air Force Medical Operations Agency/SGOC
Office of the Surgeon General
Washington, DC

The Clinical Quality Management Division of the Air Force Medical Operations Agency is responsible for oversight of clinical issues pertaining to quality improvement, licensure, credentialing and privileging, and risk management for the Air Force Surgeon General.

Air Force licensure policy is consistent with that of the Department of Defense (DOD). Air Force Medical Service physicians (military, civil service, contract personnel, and volunteers) must possess a current, valid, and unrestricted license from an official agency of a state; the District of Columbia; or a commonwealth, territory, or possession of the United States to provide health care independently within the scope of the license. Physicians must have a medical license that meets all clinical, professional, and administrative requirements of the issuing state and be no different than that of civilian counterparts.

Personnel accessed from professional training or who complete other training and require a license must obtain such license within 1 year of the date when all required didactic and clinical requirements are met, or within 1 year of completion of graduate year one. Physicians who do not yet meet licensure requirements may practice only under a written plan of supervision by a licensed, fully qualified, independently practicing, privileged provider of same or similar specialty. The Air Force requires physicians who choose to be licensed in a state that requires more than 1 year of graduate training to first obtain a license from a state that requires only 1 year of graduate training.

Department of the Army

Howard M. Kimes, Colonel, US Army
Director, Quality Management Directorate

Janet L. Wilson, Lieutenant Colonel, US Army
Chief, Regulatory Compliance
US Army Medical Command
Fort Sam Houston, Texas

The US Army Medical Command's Quality Management Directorate is responsible for developing policy and overseeing all facets of the Army Surgeon General's Quality Assurance Program, including quality improvement, credentials review and privileging, licensure, and risk management. The Directorate serves as the conduit for issues concerning clinical standards and accreditation by the Joint Commission for Accreditation of Healthcare Organizations for US Army Medicine Worldwide.

Department of Defense physicians (military and civilian, contractors and partners) must possess a current valid, unrestricted license from an official agency of the District of Columbia or a state, commonwealth, territory, or possession of the United States to provide health care independently within the scope of their licenses. Physicians in graduate medical education (GME) programs must possess a license within 1 year from the completion of their first year of GME training. An exception exists for individuals who complete their first year of GME in a state requiring 2 or more years of GME for licensure and who are assigned with that same state. These individuals must possess a license within 1 year of completion of their second year of GME training.

Healthcare providers awaiting a required license work only under the supervision of a licensed provider.

Department of the Navy

Morgan Sammons, Captain,
Medical Service Corps, US Navy
Director, Clinical Operations
Bureau of Medicine and Surgery
Department of the Navy
Washington, DC

Georgi Irvine, Commander, Nurse Corps, US Navy (Ret)
Head, Medical and Dental Staff Services
Navy Medical Support Command
Jacksonville, Florida

The Clinical Operations Division within the Bureau of Medicine and Surgery, Department of the Navy (DON), is responsible for developing policy and directing the development and implementation of US Navy-wide quality management and professional affairs programs to improve the quality of patient care; reduce risks to our customers, guests, and staff; advance good stewardship; and maintain accreditation by the Joint Commission for Accreditation of Healthcare Organizations of all US Navy fixed medical treatment facilities.

Federal regulations require physicians and other health providers within the military health services system to possess a professional license or certification. The DON further requires the license to be current, valid, unrestricted, and one to which quality management data accrues. All DON physicians (military, civilian, civilian contract, and partnership), except interns, must possess a license from a recognized, official agency of a state; the District of Columbia; or a commonwealth, territory, or possession of the United States to provide health care services independently within the scope of their license. Licenses issued by authorities allowing reduced or no fees for military personnel must meet the same licensure criteria. Health care practitioners lacking required license or certification may work only under a plan of supervision with a licensed practitioner of the same or a similar professional discipline. This policy supports the US Navy's goal to ensure all practitioners are available for worldwide assignment and rapid deployment.

Federal Controlled Substances Registration

Office of Diversion Control
Drug Enforcement Administration
Washington, DC

The Controlled Substances Act of 1970 mandates that controlled substances be maintained in a "closed system of distribution" that tracks all phases of manufacture, distribution, and dispensing. The Department of Justice, through the Drug Enforcement Administration (DEA), has the responsibility to ensure the availability of controlled substances for legitimate need while preventing their diversion into illicit markets.

The Controlled Substances Act and its implementing regulations require that any person desiring to legally manufacture, distribute, or dispense controlled substances must register with the DEA. After approval, each applicant is assigned a registration number, which must be used in every transaction involving controlled substances. Use of the DEA registration number, together with required records of transactions, allows tracking of controlled substances from the point of manufacture to the point at which they are dispensed to the patient.

As of April 2006, there were 1,217,905 active DEA registrants. Practitioners account for 1,004,411 of those registrants, with an additional 47,037 new applications for registration received each year.

A physician who seeks to become registered with the DEA must submit an Application for Registration (DEA Form-224). There are several means of submitting an application.

A. Online

Application forms are available on the DEA Diversion Control Program Web site at www.DEAdiversion.usdoj.gov. Both the new application (DEA Form-224) and the renewal form (DEA Form-224a) may be completed online in one of the following ways:

1. Applications may be completed and submitted via DEA's "Office of Diversion Control Web Interactive Forms (ODWIF)." Physicians will need a browser that supports 128-bit encryption, and they must have their Tax ID and/or Social Security Number; State Controlled Substance Registration Information; State Medical License Information; and a credit card (American Express, Discover, Visa, or MasterCard) to complete the transaction. This transaction takes approximately 5 minutes and is transmitted to DEA HQ in a secure and encrypted manner.
2. Applications may be also completed in a partially interactive form in Adobe Acrobat PDF format online, where the registrant fills in the information then prints, signs, and mails the printed form to the below address.
3. Blank applications may be printed from the DEA's Web site and then filled out manually by the registrant, signed, and mailed to the below address.

B. Application Paper Form

The form can be obtained from DEA by calling the Registration Unit at 800 882-9539 or contacting a DEA field office with a registration assistant. The completed paper application (DEA Form-224) and the required fee must be mailed to:

Drug Enforcement Administration
Central Station
PO Box 530295
Atlanta, GA 30348-0295

Following initial processing by the Registration Unit, the application is referred to the appropriate DEA field office for completion after verification of controlled substances authority with the state. The application is approved and a certificate bearing the practitioner's DEA registration number is issued. This process normally takes from 4 to 6 weeks to complete. (Renewal applications generally are processed within 4 weeks.) The online new application takes approximately 5 days till a registration certification is mailed. If there are no changes from the previous registration, online renewals are mailed the following day. The DEA certificate must be maintained at the registered location and must be kept available for official inspection.

The DEA also registers practitioners who have been granted limited authority by the appropriate state licensing agency to handle controlled substances. These individuals are registered as mid-level practitioners (MLPs). As of

April 2006, 121,157 MLPs, including nurse practitioners, certified nurse-midwives, physician assistants, and optometrists, were registered with the DEA.

The fee for both new and renewal applications for all practitioners is currently $390 for a 3-year period. An exemption from payment of the application fee is provided to federal, state, or local government registrants. On November 16, 2005, the DEA published a Notice of Proposed Rule Making in the *Federal Register* (Volume 70, Number 220, pages 69474-69486) to increase the fee to $573 for a 3-year period.

A renewal application, DEA Form 224a, is mailed to each registrant approximately 60 days prior to the expiration date. Registrants who do not receive the form within 45 days prior to the expiration of their registration should contact a DEA office with a registration assistant to request a renewal application. DEA registrations are issued for controlled substances activities at specific locations. If a physician has more than one office where controlled substances will be stored, a separate registration must be obtained for each location. If the activities at a secondary location are limited to prescribing within the same state, then separate registration is not required.

The following registration information is provided:

1. When submitting a new or renewal application, or requesting a modification of a registration, allow 4 weeks for processing; DEA receives more than 35,000 requests per month.
2. One of the primary criteria for issuing a DEA registration is that the applicant be authorized by the state in which he or she will practice. Make sure that all applications for state licensing have been completed before submitting your application for DEA registration. The same applies for registrants relocating from one state to another.
3. Keep track of the expiration date of your DEA registration. Renewal notices are mailed to registrants approximately 60 days prior to expiration. If you do not receive a renewal application within 45 days prior to the expiration of your registration, call 800 882-9539. If a registration expires, the registrant is no longer authorized to handle controlled substances. Until the registration is renewed and a new certificate of registration is issued, use of the registration is a violation of the law.
4. As noted earlier, DEA registrations are issued for controlled substances activities at a specific location. Federal regulations require that DEA be notified in advance of any change of address. Additionally, the registration address cannot be a post office box. It must be the physical location where the controlled substance activities occur.
5. The Registration Unit can be contacted toll-free at 800 882-9539. Whenever contacting the DEA regarding an existing registration, provide the DEA registration number.

The DEA's registration program plays an integral role in efforts to prevent the diversion of legitimately produced controlled substances to the illicit market. The program has grown in complexity with the addition of new controlled substances as well as with new automated initiatives. The continued success of the program is the result of the combined efforts and understanding of health care professionals, industry, and the DEA.

The answers to many registration questions and the locations of DEA field offices and registration assistants are listed on the Diversion Control Program Web site, available at www.DEAdiversion.usdoj.gov.

National Practitioner Data Bank and Healthcare Integrity and Protection Data Bank

These two federal programs collect specific data nationwide about health care practitioners, providers, and suppliers.

The National Practitioner Data Bank (NPDB) collects and releases information on physicians' medical malpractice payments, adverse licensure actions, adverse clinical privilege actions, adverse professional society membership actions, and exclusions from participation in Medicare and Medicaid. The NPDB is a flagging system that facilitates a comprehensive review of actions affecting health care practitioners' professional credentials. Hospitals, managed care organizations, other authorized health care entities, professional societies, and state licensing boards use NPDB information, in conjunction with other sources, when granting clinical privileges or when making employment, affiliation, or licensure decisions. Hospitals, professional societies, and other health care organizations are also required to report certain data to the NPDB. Malpractice insurers must report all payments made for individual practitioners.

The Healthcare Integrity and Protection Data Bank (HIPDB) collects and releases information on health care practitioners, providers, and suppliers' licensure and certification actions, exclusions from participation in federal and state health care programs, criminal convictions and civil judgments related to health care, and other adjudicated actions or decisions. The HIPDB is an alert or flagging system that assists federal and state agencies, state licensing boards, and health plans in conducting extensive, independent investigations of the qualifications of health care practitioners, providers, or suppliers whom they seek to license, hire, or credential, or with whom they seek to contract or affiliate. Health plans and federal and state government agencies are required to report certain data to the HIPDB.

Both Data Banks are operated under the direct supervision of the Practitioner Data Banks Branch, Office of Workforce Evaluation and Quality Assurance, Bureau of Health Professions, Health Resources and Services Administration, US Department of Health and Human Services (HHS), although the HHS Office of the Inspector General has statutory responsibility for the HIPDB. The NPDB began collecting and disseminating information in 1990. The HIPDB began collecting information in 1999 and disseminating it in 2000.

Data Availability and Confidentiality

Information reported to the NPDB and HIPDB is considered confidential. NPDB information is available only to state licensing boards; hospitals and other health care entities, including professional societies; and others as specified in the law. HIPDB information is available only to health plans and federal and state government agencies. Information that identifies individuals is not available to the general public. Statistical information is made available to the public.

Health care practitioners, providers, and suppliers are allowed to query their own records in the NPDB and HIPDB at any time. All self-query requests are automatically sent to both Data Banks, and a fee of $8 is assessed by each Data Bank. A self-query may not be sent to only one Data Bank. Subjects of a report in either Data Bank receive with their self-query responses a list of all parties to whom the report has been disclosed. To self-query, see: www.npdb-hipdb.hrsa.gov/welcomesq.html

Reporting, Statements, and Disputing Reports

NPDB and HIPDB reporting and querying are done electronically through a secure Internet site, at www.npdb-hipdb.hrsa.gov. Reporting is combined, with a set of rules determining how reports are accepted into each Data Bank. Based on the information submitted, the NPDB-HIPDB computer system routes reports to the appropriate Data Bank(s). Queriers eligible for both Data Banks may also submit one query that is routed to both.

After processing a report from a reporting entity, the NPDB and HIPDB sends a notice to the entity and to the individual or organizations ("subjects") mentioned in the report. If there are errors, subjects must ask the reporting entity to correct the information. Both Data Banks are prohibited from modifying information submitted in reports except through a "Secretarial Review" process established to resolve disputed reports not corrected by the reporting entities.

Subjects of a NPDB or HIPDB report may add a statement to the report, dispute either the factual accuracy of the information in a report or whether the report was submitted in accordance with NPDB or HIPDB reporting requirements, or both. If the reporting entity does not make a correction satisfactory to the subject of a report, the subject may request "Secretarial Review." The HHS will then review whether the report was legally filed and accurate.

Responsibilities of State Boards

State licensing boards must report to the NPDB certain adverse licensure actions related to professional competence or professional conduct and any changes to such actions. These actions include revocation, suspension, censure, reprimand, probation, and surrender. Boards must also report revisions to adverse licensure actions. State boards must report to the HIPDB final adverse actions taken against health care practitioners, providers, or suppliers.

Available Materials

Materials available from the Data Banks include the National Practitioner Data Bank *Guidebook*; Healthcare Integrity and Protection Data Bank *Guidebook*; fact sheets on various topics; and self-query materials. All of the materials are available on the Internet at www.npdb-hipdb.hrsa.gov.

National Practitioner Data Bank and
Healthcare Integrity and Protection Data Bank
PO Box 10832
Chantilly, VA 20151
800 767-6732
www.npdb-hipdb.hrsa.gov

Section VI.

Other Organizations and Programs

American Board of Medical Specialties

The American Board of Medical Specialties (ABMS®), a not-for-profit organization, represents 24 approved medical specialty boards that establish and maintain high standards for physician certification and the delivery of safe, quality medical care by certified physician specialists. The primary function of the ABMS is to assist the Member Boards in their efforts to develop and use standards for the evaluation and certification of physician specialists.

Additionally, in collaboration with other organizations and the Accreditation Council for Graduate Medical Education (ACGME), the Member Boards assist in improving the quality of medical education by elevating the standards for graduate medical education and accreditation (approval) of residency and training programs.

The ABMS Member Boards (listed below) have been approved by the ABMS and the AMA Council on Medical Education (AMA CME) through the Liaison Committee for Specialty Boards (LCSB), with ultimate approval of the application by the membership of the ABMS and the AMA CME.

American Board of:

- Allergy and Immunology
- Anesthesiology
- Colon and Rectal Surgery
- Dermatology
- Emergency Medicine
- Family Medicine
- Internal Medicine
- Medical Genetics
- Neurological Surgery
- Nuclear Medicine
- Obstetrics and Gynecology
- Ophthalmology
- Orthopaedic Surgery
- Otolaryngology
- Pathology
- Pediatrics
- Physical Medicine and Rehabilitation
- Plastic Surgery
- Preventive Medicine
- Psychiatry and Neurology
- Radiology
- Surgery
- Thoracic Surgery
- Urology

The governing body of each ABMS Member Board is composed of specialists qualified in the particular field represented by that board. They are elected to the board from national specialty organizations in fields related to the particular specialty involved. These individuals can include teachers in the specialty, those with specialized training or skills in the primary specialty or subspecialties represented by the Board, and from among those who have demonstrated the expertise, motivation, and ability to assist in the evaluation procedures leading to certification.

About Specialties in Medicine

Specialties in medicine develop because of the rapidly expanding body of knowledge about health and illness and the constantly evolving treatment techniques for disease. Some specialists are primary care doctors, such as family physicians, general internists, and general pediatricians. Other specialists concentrate on certain body systems, specific age groups, or complex scientific techniques developed to diagnose or treat certain types of disorders.

A subspecialist is a physician who has completed training in a general medical/surgical specialty and takes additional training in a more specific area of that specialty called a subspecialty. This training increases the depth of knowledge and expertise of the specialist in that particular field.

Specialty Board Certification and Medical Licensure

To better understand the importance of certification, one must first understand the differences between licensure and certification.

Medical licensure provides a physician with the legal privilege to practice medicine. It is not specialty-specific or designed to recognize the knowledge and skills of a trained specialist, but a legal necessity, granted by state governments, that permits a physician to take on personal and unsupervised responsibility for the diagnosis and treatment of patients in the broad practice of medicine.

Licensure establishes the minimum competence that is essential to protecting the health, safety, and welfare of the public. A physician is granted a license to practice by a state board of medical examiners after completing a certain amount of training and passing a national, and in a few instances a state, licensure examination. Each state or territory has its own procedures to license physicians and sets the general standards for all physicians in that state or territory.

Certification of physician specialists, a practice which has existed for nearly 90 years, is separate from medical licensure and has largely been voluntary. However, with the current forces affecting health care, more and more physicians are being required or are electing to seek formal recognition of their qualifications.

Certification obtained through one of the ABMS Member Boards denotes that a physician has gone beyond the minimum requirement necessary for licensure. It provides the assurance that a physician has the appropriate knowledge, skills, and experience needed to deliver quality care in a specific area of medicine according to the standards designated by the ABMS and its Member Boards.

The ABMS Member Boards oversee the certification process for their particular specialty. A physician receives certification as a specialty medical practitioner after completing an accredited training program, undergoing an evaluation of his or her record by a panel of peer experts, and passing a comprehensive examination given by an ABMS Member Board.

Physicians meeting this set of requirements are awarded general certificates in the field represented by that Member Board. Physicians can also become certified in a subspecialty, a particular area within the specialty, which requires additional training and examination.

Continuous Certification of Physician Specialists

Recognizing that the professional responsibility of physicians requires ongoing learning and improvement throughout their careers, a program of continuous certification called Maintenance of Certification (MOC) was developed by the ABMS and the Member Boards as a formal means of measuring a physician's cumulative and ongoing qualifications in the specialty and/or subspecialty in which certification is held.

With the MOC program, the ABMS Member Boards are moving away from periodic (every 6, 7, or 10 years) recertification by examination to a more comprehensive process for assessing the continuing competence of physician specialists and their ability to provide quality health care. The MOC processes assure that the physician is maintaining an appropriate level of knowledge in the specialty to promote optimal health outcomes.

The MOC program incorporates the latest research on physician competence, patient safety, and practice management care and focuses on six general competencies:

- Patient care
- Medical knowledge
- Practice-based learning and improvement
- Interpersonal and communications skills
- Professionalism
- Systems-based practice

These areas were identified jointly by the ABMS and the ACGME as those which are crucial for a physician to deliver high-quality patient care.

MOC was initially proposed in 1998-99 and developed with the involvement of a broad spectrum of medical and surgical specialties. The effort is supported by many major medical organizations, including the:

- American Medical Association (AMA)
- American Hospital Association (AHA)
- National Board of Medical Examiners (NBME)

- Federation of State Medical Boards of the US (FSMB)
- Joint Commission on Accreditation of Healthcare Organizations (JCAHO)
- Council of Medical Specialty Societies (CMSS)
- Accreditation Council for Graduate Medical Education (ACGME)
- Association of American Medical Colleges (AAMC)
- Educational Commission for Foreign Medical Graduates (ECFMG).

The MOC process has four basic components:

1. Professional standing
Documents that the certified physician has met and maintains legal requirements to practice medicine. All licenses held by a physician must be unrestricted.

2. Lifelong learning and self-assessment
This component enables physicians to reaffirm their commitment to continuous learning and improvement and to assume a leadership role in the quest for safe, quality health care. This requires evidence of participation in educational and self-assessment programs and meeting specialty-specific standards. It is integrated with practice performance to provide a real world practice basis to guide learning and enables physicians to put their learning to use continuously and regularly in the process of normal patient care.

3. Cognitive expertise
Provides evidence, through an examination, that physician specialists have the necessary knowledge to provide quality patient care. Examinations cover the scope and range of the discipline and are clinically relevant.

4. Practice performance assessment
This component focuses on improvement in the quality of care through collaborative efforts with other organizations. Physicians are evaluated in their clinical practice according to specialty-specific standards for patient care. They are provided with feedback and techniques for improvement.

Verifying Physician Certification

For all except those recently certified as specialists by an ABMS Member Board, and not yet entered into the ABMS certification database, and except for a very small number of specialists who do not wish to be listed, the fact of certification may be determined through these public services:

- The Who's Certified service on the ABMS Web site (www.abms.org)
- The ABMS's toll-free Physician Verification service at 866-ASK-ABMS
- The *Official ABMS Directory of Certified Medical Specialists*® available in most public libraries

These resources are not valid for accrediting done by credentialing organizations or other commercial entities. Groups that perform mass verifications must obtain their information from a recognized source, such as the ABMS, or an ABMS-designated agent. ABMS offers a number of verification services to the medical staff and credentialing professionals and other business users.

For more information about the ABMS, ABMS member boards, the certification of physician specialists, and verifying physician certification, contact:

American Board of Medical Specialties
1007 Church St, Ste 404
Evanston, IL 60201-5913
847 491-9091
847 328-3596 Fax
www.abms.org

Accreditation Council for Graduate Medical Education

The Accreditation Council for Graduate Medical Education (ACGME) is an accrediting agency composed of directors nominated by five national associations interested in graduate medical education: the American Board of Medical Specialties, American Hospital Association, American Medical Association, Association of American Medical Colleges, and Council of Medical Specialty Societies.

The federal government names a representative to serve in a nonvoting capacity, and the ACGME chooses three public directors. There are also two voting resident physicians: a resident director nominated by the Resident and Fellow Section of the AMA, with the advice of other national organizations that represent residents, and the chair of the Council of Review Committee Chairs.

A Residency Review Committee (RRC) consists of representatives appointed by the AMA, the appropriate specialty board, and, in some cases, a national specialty organization. The Transitional Year Review Committee is composed of nine members who are appointed by the chair of the ACGME in conjunction with the Executive Committee. The term *review committee* is used to denote a Residency Review Committee, Transitional Year Review Committee, or Institutional Review Committee.

GME programs are accredited by the appropriate review committee through authority delegated by the ACGME. Accreditation of a residency program indicates that it is judged to be in substantial compliance with the program requirements for residency education in the particular specialty.

A list of programs accredited by the ACGME, including detailed information about each program, is published annually by the AMA in the *Graduate Medical Education Directory.* The most current listing can be found on the ACGME Web site at www.acgme.org.

ACGME General Competencies

In 1999, the ACGME endorsed General Competencies in the following six areas. ACGME Program Requirements state that GME programs must define the specific knowledge, skills, and attitudes required and provide educational experiences as needed in order for their residents/fellows to demonstrate these competencies to the level expected of a new practitioner.

Patient Care that is compassionate, appropriate, and effective for the treatment of health problems and the promotion of health

Medical Knowledge about established and evolving biomedical, clinical, and cognate (eg, epidemiological and social-behavioral) sciences and the application of this knowledge to patient care

Practice-Based Learning and Improvement that involves investigation and evaluation of their own patient care, appraisal and assimilation of scientific evidence, and improvements in patient care

Interpersonal and Communication Skills that result in effective information exchange and teaming with patients, their families, and other health professionals

Professionalism, as manifested through a commitment to carrying out professional responsibilities, adherence to ethical principles, and sensitivity to a diverse patient population

Systems-Based Practice, as manifested by actions that demonstrate an awareness of and responsiveness to the larger context and system of health care and the ability to effectively call on system resources to provide care of optimal value

Contact Information

Accreditation Council for Graduate Medical Education
515 N State St, 20th Fl
Chicago, IL 60610
312 755-5000
312 755-7498 Fax
www.acgme.org

American Medical Association Survey and Data Resources

The AMA Division of Survey and Data Resources is dedicated to effectively and accurately collecting, analyzing, and managing physician data within the Physician Masterfile. The AMA Physician Masterfile is a data source not only for internal use but also for use by other professional medical organizations, universities and medical schools, research institutions, governmental agencies, and other related groups. The use of Physician Masterfile data by agencies and organizations concerned with verifying physicians' credentials and health manpower planning is fundamental to the AMA's mission to strengthen the medical profession and ensure quality health care for the American public.

The Physician Masterfile comprises a database of current and historical data on more than 820,000 physicians in the United States, both AMA members and nonmembers. This figure includes approximately 210,000 graduates of foreign medical schools who reside in the United States and who have met the educational and credentialing requirements necessary for recognition and approximately 50,000 doctors of osteopathy. Physician records are never removed from the AMA Physician Masterfile. Records of deceased physicians are shared with other organizations and are used to identify individuals who fraudulently attempt to assume the credentials of deceased physicians.

Survey and Data Resources is composed of two departments:

- Census and Self-Reported Data
- Primary Source Physician Data

These departments are essential in maintaining the Masterfile as one of the most comprehensive and accurate sources of physician data.

Census and Self-Reported Data

The responsibility of this department is to track physicians throughout their training and professional careers and to collect and maintain the most accurate practice and communications data. The Department of Census and Self-Reported Data is responsible for collecting program and individual resident data from approximately 8,400 residency/fellowship training programs via the annual National GME Census, collecting communications and practice information from up to 250,000 physicians annually via the Census of Physicians, updating more than 300,000 physician mailing addresses per year, and collecting roster information annually from more than 45,000 medical group locations maintained on the AMA's Group Practice Database.

One of the main functions of the Census and Self-Reported Data department is the processing of resident information collected via the National GME Census. This is an online survey that is conducted in a joint effort with the Association of American Medical Colleges (AAMC). Each year, approximately 8,200 ACGME-accredited and 200 ABMS Board-approved GME programs are surveyed. The reported residency information is internally validated and incorporated into a physician's record. The survey also includes questions on GME program characteristics, such as clinical and research facilities and the learning environment, which are used to update FREIDA Online® (www.ama-assn.org/go/freida) and the *Graduate Medical Education Directory*, produced by the Division of Graduate Medical Education.

Once physicians complete residency and/or fellowship training, the Census and Self-Reported Data department tracks physicians throughout their professional careers. The annual Census of Physicians, for example, surveys approximately 250,000 physicians per year and collects information on a physician's professional medical activities, preferred mailing address, principal hospital and group affiliations, and practice specialties, among other data. This unit also utilizes over 15 additional sources to supplement data collected via the Physicians Census. The information that is captured is used to support membership efforts, communicate with physicians, segment physician markets, draw samples for health-related research, and track professional trends.

Another function of this unit is to maintain preferred professional mailing address information for the Physician Masterfile. Each year, approximately 300,000 physician addresses are updated from over 20 sources. To ensure high-quality and deliverable addresses, the AMA also subscribes to the USPS Address Correction System (ACS) from which it receives weekly address updates, and uses the US Postal Service's National Change of Address (NCOA) Service and the Delivery Sequence File (DSF) Service on a quarterly basis.

The Census and Self-Reported Data department also surveys medical group practices in order to maintain the Group Practice Database. This database contains information and affiliations for more than 45,000 group practice locations. These data are mainly used for membership development and marketing products and services.

Primary Source Physician Data

The responsibility of the Department of Primary Source Physician Data is to procure and process data obtained from primary source organizations such as medical schools, licensing authorities, medical specialty boards, etc. It is within this department that each individual AMA Physician Masterfile record is first established. This occurs when individuals enter medical school programs accredited by the Liaison Committee on Medical Education (LCME) in the United States or Canada. In the case of international medical graduates (IMGs), a record is established upon entry into residency programs accredited by the Accreditation Council for Graduate Medical Education (ACGME). Background information on these individuals is verified with the Educational Commission for Foreign Medical Graduates (ECFMG). Doctors of osteopathy are added to the Masterfile through AMA annual surveys and membership solicitations or through the processing of new licensure data as reported by state licensing authorities.

As new records are created, a record identifier called the Medical Education (ME) number is assigned. This number remains the same throughout a physician's medical career. Physician records are never removed from the Masterfile, even in the case of death.

The department procures and processes over 34 million updates annually from the 68 state medical and osteopathic jurisdictions that license physicians. Monthly updates are also procured from the US Department of Justice Drug Enforcement Administration, updating controlled substance registration information for more than 700,000 physician records, and the American Board of Medical Specialties, updating physician board certification data. Other primary sources include medical school data obtained in concert with the Association of American Medical Colleges and data on IMGs as reported by the ECFMG.

Processing of Primary Source Physician Data involves a system called CAM (Computer Assisted Matching) that is used to match the ME number to other numerically based information, such as state license or board certification number. This system helps in processing the millions of records processed each year by the department.

In order to procure primary source data, this department must build and maintain data exchange relationships, so that the AMA continues to obtain and manage valuable physician information. The unit serves as a liaison with outside organizations from which it receives data (eg, licensing jurisdictions, certifying agencies, and professional associations). A major function of the Department of Primary Source Physician Data is to collect physician licensure and disciplinary action data. For many years the AMA has collected active and historical licensure data from the 68 jurisdictions that license physicians. In 1997, the AMA expanded its procurement activities to include physician disciplinary data. To date all US state licensing jurisdictions, the US Department of Health and Human Services, and the US Department of Justice Drug Enforcement Administration have reported physician disciplinary with much of the information spanning as far back as a decade. The AMA has received nationwide recognition as the only entity that maintains a complete history of physician-specific licensure activity across allopathic and osteopathic state licensing authorities.

Data Quality and Measurement

Data Quality and Measurement is a business unit within the Department of Primary Source Physician Data. The responsibilities of this unit are to **educate** others about the Physician Masterfile, **facilitate** access to the Physician Masterfile, and **evaluate** the quality of the Physician Masterfile.

Data Quality and Measurement **educates** data users about the Physician Masterfile by

- Maintaining the Physician Data Resources pages on the AMA's Web site, available at www.ama-assn.org/ama/pub/category/2670.html

- Managing and responding to telephone, email and written inquiries regarding Masterfile data from existing and potential customers
- Planning and coordinating the preparation and maintenance of process documentation

Data Quality and Measurement **facilitates** access to the Physician Masterfile by

- Fulfilling more than 500 data requests a year that support the communications, marketing, and planning efforts of other AMA units
- Publishing aggregate statistics on the physician population in *Physician Characteristics and Distribution in the US*
- Managing the AMA's corporate mailing list application, which includes more than 100 different list directories and supports key Association activities involving the AMA board, councils, committees, advisory groups, and House of Delegates
- Publishing the Federation and Pictorial Directories on the AMA Web site
- Providing a mechanism and data resources for use by medical schools, universities, research institutions, governmental agencies, and other organizations interested in the study of heath care policy issues
- Coordinating the distribution of Masterfile-related reports, physician profiles, and data to state, county, and national specialty medical societies
- Coordinating the online data collection center submissions

Data Quality and Measurement **evaluates** the quality of the Physician Masterfile by

- Conducting validation studies
- Developing, measuring, and monitoring key performance indicators
- Investigating, verifying, and resolving data anomalies reported by customers, members, and others with primary source data providers
- Identifying, researching, and analyzing potential new sources of data as well as new tools to enhance data processing

Contact Information

Division of Survey and Data Resources
Monica Quiroz, Director
312 464-4153
monica.quiroz@ama-assn.org

Department of Census and Self-Reported Data
Susan Montrimas, Director
312 464-5184
susan.montrimas@ama-assn.org

American Medical Association Continuing Medical Education

Advances in biomedical science and changes in the other facets of the US health care delivery environment engage physicians in a continuous process of professional development. To ensure that they provide patients with the most current and appropriate treatment, services, and information, physicians keep learning through participation in a wide array of conferences and other teaching experiences, as well as through independent study of published materials. The American Medical Association (AMA) supports these physician efforts by engaging in the following:

- Administering the only non-specialty-specific credit system that recognizes physician completion of continuing medical education (CME) activities
- Offering CME publications and activities (both live and enduring materials, such as monographs and course materials)
- Establishing new learning modalities (eg, performance improvement and Internet point of care) appropriate for physician professional development and investigating international opportunities for reciprocal CME relationships

The AMA Physician's Recognition Award

In 1968, the AMA House of Delegates established the AMA Physician's Recognition Award (PRA) to both encourage physicians to participate in CME and acknowledge when individual physicians complete CME activities. Activities that meet education standards established by the AMA can be designated *AMA PRA Category 1 Credit*™ by educational institutions accredited to provide CME to physicians. These typically include state medical societies, medical specialty societies, medical schools, and hospitals. Other activities, usually independent or physician directed learning, may be reported for *AMA PRA Category 2 Credit*™.

AMA PRA certificates are awarded in lengths of 1, 2, or 3 years, with the following requirements:

1-year certificate – 50 credits
- 20 credits Category 1
- 30 credits Category 1 or 2

2-year certificate – 100 credits
- 40 credits Category 1
- 60 credits Category 1 or 2

3-year certificate – 150 credits
- 60 credits Category 1
- 90 credits Category 1 or 2

The AMA also offers the PRA with Commendation, awarded to physicians who exceed the credit required to earn the regular PRA. For more information, visit www.ama-assn.org/go/pra.

Through reciprocity arrangements, the AMA will also award the PRA certificate if the CME requirements of the following organizations are met:

- American Academy of Dermatology
- American Academy of Family Physicians
- American Academy of Ophthalmology
- American Academy of Otolaryngology — Head and Neck Surgery
- American Academy of Pediatrics
- American College of Emergency Physicians
- American College of Obstetricians and Gynecologists
- American College of Preventive Medicine
- American Psychiatric Association
- American Society of Clinical Pathologists/ College of American Pathologists
- American Society of Plastic Surgeons
- American Urological Association Education and Research, Inc
- California Medical Association
- Medical Society of New Jersey
- National Medical Association

The following states accept the PRA certificate as evidence that physicians have met the CME requirements for license (MD board unless otherwise noted):

- Alaska
- Arkansas
- California (MD/DO)
- Delaware
- Florida
- Guam
- Hawaii
- Idaho
- Illinois
- Kansas
- Kentucky
- Louisiana
- Maine (MD/DO)
- Maryland
- Massachusetts
- Minnesota
- Nebraska
- Nevada (MD/DO)
- New Hampshire
- New Mexico (MD/DO)
- North Dakota
- Ohio
- Oklahoma
- Pennsylvania
- Puerto Rico
- Rhode Island
- Tennessee
- Texas
- Utah
- Vermont (DO)
- Virgin Islands
- Washington (MD/DO)
- West Virginia
- Wisconsin
- Wyoming

In addition, the following states accept an AMA-approved, original AMA PRA certificate application for licensure:

- Arizona
- Iowa
- Mississippi

The Joint Commission on Accreditation of Healthcare Organizations (JCAHO) will accept, subject to review, correctly completed AMA PRA applications stamped "approved" by the AMA as documented physician compliance with JCAHO CME requirements.

The AMA sends PRA application forms to physicians who have had a valid PRA certificate within the past 3 years and physicians whose current certificate is expiring within 3 months. The AMA PRA application form and the PRA Information Booklet, respectively, are available online at

www.ama-assn.org/go/applypra
www.ama-assn.org/go/prabooklet

or by contacting:

Department of Accreditation and Certification Activities
Continuing Physician Professional Development
American Medical Association
515 N State St
Chicago, IL 60610
312 464-4941
312 464-4567 Fax
E-mail: pra@ama-assn.org

For bulk orders of the AMA Physician's Recognition Award Booklet, contact the AMA Order Department at 800 621-8335.

AMA CME Programs

Enduring (Self-Assessment) CME Programs

The AMA Healthcare Education Products and Standards Group offers a number of enduring CME programs that provide physician self-assessment. These programs offer quality CME in a convenient format that permits learners to work at their own pace and at a time that fits a busy clinical schedule. Available in print, CD-ROM, and Internet formats, these enduring CME programs are dedicated to improving the effectiveness and scope of CME programs by exploring new formats and delivery approaches that tap into the latest clinical information and that meet the AMA's rigorous CME standards. An updated list of available programs can be accessed at www.ama-cme.org, and many Internet programs allow physicians to print their own CME certificates.

Monographs/Internet Programs

The AMA Healthcare Education Products and Standards Group produces and distributes both printed self-study monographs and Internet/CD-ROM programs, which are developed in cooperation with medical specialty societies and recognized medical experts and funded with educational grant support from industry. These programs are intended for primary care physicians and interested medical specialists. Programs are available in the areas shown in Table 34.

Table 34
CME Products Available From AMA Healthcare Education Products and Standards

Area	Program Title	CME Credits	Availability		
			Print	Internet	pdf
Genetics	Risk Assessment for Hereditary Cancer Syndromes: A Physician's Guide to Clinical Genetic Testing and Medical Management	3	X		X
Hepatitis C Virus	Update on the Screening and Management of HCV Infection in Adults	3	X		
Immunization	A Focus on Immunization and Preventable Disease Management	2		X	X
Neurological Conditions	Pain Management: The Online Series				
	Module 1: Pathophysiology of Pain and Pain Assessment	1		X	
	Module 2: Overview of Management Options	1		X	
	Module 3: Barriers to Pain Management and Pain in Special Populations	1		X	
	Module 4: Assessing and Treating Pain in Patients with Substance Abuse Concerns	1		X	
	Module 5: Assessing and Treating Pain in Older Adults	1		X	
	Module 6: Pediatric Pain Management	1		X	
	Module 7: Assessing and Treating Persistent Nonmalignant Pain - An Overview	1		X	
	Module 8: Common Persistent Pain Conditions	1		X	
	Module 9: Assessing and Treating Neuropathic Pain	1		X	
	Module 10: Overview and Assessment of Cancer Pain	1		X	
	Module 11: Cancer Pain Pharmacotherapy	1		X	
	Module 12: Management of Cancer Pain—Other Analgesic Approaches and End-of-Life Care	1		X	
Osteoporosis	Managing Osteoporosis: The Online Series				
	Introduction, Obstacles, Assessing Risk Factors	1.5		X	
	Recommendations for BMD Measurement and Techniques for Testing	1.5		X	
	Pathophysiology of Osteoporosis	1.5		X	
	Nonpharmacologic Prevention and Treatment of Osteoporosis	1.5		X	
	Pharmacologic Prevention and Treatment of Osteoporosis	1.5		X	
	Treatment of Postmenopausal Osteoporosis	1.5		X	
	Osteoporosis in Men	1.5		X	
	Glucocorticoid-Induced Osteoporosis	1.5		X	
	Rehabilitation of the Patient with Osteoporosis	1.5		X	
	Postmenopausal Osteoporosis: Case Study of 56 Year-Old Woman	1.5		X	
	Postmenopausal Osteoporosis: Case Study of 60 Year-Old Woman Discontinuing HT	1.5		X	
	Male Osteoporosis: Case Study of 70 Year-Old Man Receiving Androgen-Deprivation Therapy	1.5		X	
	State-of-the-Art Management of Osteoporosis	4	X		
Pain Management	Part 1: Overview of Physiology, Assessment and Treatment	3	X		X
	Part 2: Assessing and Treating Pain in Special Populations	3	X		X
	Part 3: Management of Persistent Nonmalignant Pain	3	X		X
	Part 4: Cancer and End-of-Life Care	3	X		X
Respiratory Diseases	Chronic Bronchitis	3	X		

Journal CME

The AMA has launched online journal CME activities for the *Journal of the American Medical Association* and in the following six AMA *Archives* journals. Physicians can earn AMA PRA Category 1 credit by reading the designated articles online and completing a post-test.

- *Archives of Dermatology*
- *Archives of Internal Medicine*
- *Archives of Neurology*
- *Archives of Ophthalmology*
- *Archives of Otolaryngology—Head and Neck Surgery*
- *Archives of Surgery*

AMA-sponsored Conferences and Live Events

As an ACCME-accredited provider, the AMA sponsors multiple conferences and live events designated for AMA PRA Category 1 credit. Physicians receive education on topics of interest to all disciplines and specialties. Recently, AMA-sponsored or cosponsored conferences and live events have included Basic and Advanced Disaster Life Support programs, the AMA Medical Communications and Health Reporting Conference, the North American Metabolic Syndrome Forum, and the Women Physician Leaders Summit.

International CME

The International Conference Recognition Program began in 1990 by an act of the AMA House of Delegates. The AMA recognized that international congresses present opportunities for physicians to participate in quality educational programs and provide opportunities for US physicians to collaborate with colleagues overseas. The AMA recognizes a handful of events each year and provides American physicians with an opportunity to earn AMA PRA Category 1 credit at these approved events. For more information, visit www.ama-assn.org/go/internationalcme.

Contact Information

For more information on AMA CME programs and activities, visit www.ama-assn.org/go/cme or contact:

Multimedia CME	312 464-5990
AMA CME credits/courses	312 464-4941
Physician's Recognition Award	312 464-4672
International CME	312 464-5196

For general information, contact:

Continuing Physician Professional Development
American Medical Association
515 N State St
Chicago, IL 60610
312 464-4671
312 464-5830 Fax
E-mail: cppd@ama-assn.org

American Medical Association Project USA

Now more than a quarter of a century old, Project USA is an American Medical Association (AMA) program that recruits physicians for short-term service in rural areas. Funded by the US Public Health Service, Project USA is a coordinated effort involving the AMA and the Indian Health Service. The purpose of the program is to provide temporary short-term replacements for Public Health Service physicians, enabling them to take vacations or fulfill continuing education requirements.

Primary care physicians with a full and unrestricted license to practice medicine are being sought to participate in Project USA. Openings are available year round for 2 to 4 weeks or longer. These locum tenens positions provide a weekly salary, malpractice insurance coverage, and round-trip coach airfare; housing accommodations are also available.

Project USA volunteers may be part of a health care team that includes dentists, nurses, and other health personnel while serving at a three- or four-doctor Indian Health Service hospital, or may work in a solo-practice setting.

The Need for Project USA

Medically underserved rural areas are in need of the continuing medical services that physicians can provide. Physicians who volunteer for Project USA have an opportunity to become exposed to totally different cultures and to find new perspectives and insights, both medical and social. They also enjoy the satisfaction that comes from responding to a need for their professional services and the appreciation of rural people for their contributions to the health care of their community.

Contact Information

John Naughton, Project Director
Project USA, American Medical Association
515 N State St
Chicago, IL 60610
312 464-4702
800 388-4702
312 464-4184 Fax
E-mail: john.naughton@ama-assn.org
www.ama-assn.org/go/projectusa

Joint Commission on Accreditation of Healthcare Organizations

An independent, nonprofit organization, the Joint Commission on Accreditation of Healthcare Organizations (JCAHO), or Joint Commission, evaluates and accredits about 15,000 health care organizations and programs in the United States and other countries. Accreditation by the Joint Commission is internationally recognized as a symbol of quality indicating that an organization meets state-of-the-art performance standards.

Joint Commission staff work with health care experts, practitioners, providers, researchers, purchasers, and consumers around the world to develop optimal achievable performance standards, all with a single focus—to improve the safety and quality of patient care.

To earn and maintain accreditation, an organization must undergo an on-site survey by a team of Joint Commission surveyors at least every 3 years (laboratories are surveyed every 2 years). These surveys are conducted on an unannounced basis. The Joint Commission employs more than 400 experienced physicians, nurses, health care administrators, medical technologists, psychologists, pharmacists, and other medical professionals to conduct these surveys.

Accreditation Programs

The Joint Commission operates the following eight accreditation programs, which serve various types of health care organizations:

- Hospital Accreditation Program
- Home Care Accreditation Program
- Ambulatory Care Accreditation Program
- Laboratory Accreditation Program
- Long-Term Care Accreditation Program
- Behavioral Health Care Accreditation Program
- Critical Access Hospital Accreditation Program

Benefits of Accreditation

Accreditation by the Joint Commission offers the following benefits:

- Assists organizations in improving the safety and quality of the care they provide
- Strengthens community confidence
- Provides professional advice and ongoing support
- Enhances staff education and recruitment
- Fulfills licensure and certification requirements in many states
- Attracts professional referrals
- Confers Medicare and Medicaid certification for some types of organizations
- Is recognized by insurers, expedites third-party payment, and may favorably influence liability insurance premiums

Major Initiatives

The Joint Commission works to improve the safety and quality of health care through such projects as the Sentinel Event Database and the ORYX initiative. The former permits dissemination of lessons learned from analysis of serious adverse events by accredited organizations and serves as the basis for the annual issuance of National Patient Safety Goals. The latter establishes performance measurement and reporting requirements and supports quality improvement efforts within accredited organizations.

In addition, the Joint Commission has a standards-based Disease-Specific Care program, which also incorporates the use of clinical practice guidelines and performance measures. Finally, accreditation services for office-based surgery are provided under the Ambulatory Care program.

The newest Joint Commission initiative has involved the convening of an ongoing series of Public Policy Roundtables. Each project culminates in a national summit and the publication of a white paper with explicit recommendations and assigned accountabilities. The white papers on the nurse staffing crisis, emergency preparedness, organ donation, and tort resolution and patient safety have received extensive national attention. Projects on emergency department overcrowding, health professions education reform, health literacy, and the hospital of the future are currently in progress.

Consumers can find information about JCAHO-accredited health care organizations online through Quality Check™, which is accessible through the Joint Commission's Web site at www.jcaho.org. Quality reports that provide detailed information about each accredited institution are also available through Quality Check.

Origins/Governance

The Joint Commission was founded in 1951. Its governing Board of Commissioners consists of 29 individuals whose backgrounds and experience reflect a broad range of professional and lay interests. The board includes practicing physicians, health care executives, nurses, and public members whose expertise includes bioethics, labor relations, business, education, and quality improvement, among others. The established reputation of the Joint Commission as a health care quality evaluator permits it direct access to a wide array of experts and public policy makers to guide it in developing and maintaining state-of-the-art standards and performance measures.

Joint Commission on Accreditation of Healthcare Organizations (JCAHO)
One Renaissance Blvd
Oakbrook Terrace, IL 60181
630 792-5000
630 792-5005 Fax
www.jcaho.org

National Association Medical Staff Services

Formed in 1978, the National Association Medical Staff Services (NAMSS) is an international association that provides professional education resources to individuals in the areas of health care credentialing, clinical privileging, practitioner/provider organizations, and regulatory compliance. Its mission is to protect and promote high-quality health care for the public by helping its members understand and succeed in the changing organizational structures of the health care industry. It also develops, administers, and promotes certification programs that measure knowledge of current industry standards and practices.

For more information, contact:

National Association Medical Staff Services
2025 M St, NW
Washington, DC 20036

Mailing address:
Dept 3115
Washington, DC 20042

202 367-1196
202 367-2196 Fax
www.namss.org

National Committee for Quality Assurance

The National Committee for Quality Assurance (NCQA) is a private, not-for-profit organizations that assesses and reports on the quality of health care services in multiple areas of the health care system in order to provide a basis for quality improvement activities and for public reporting of performance. The efforts of NCQA are organized around programs providing accreditation and certification of organizations, including health plans and other entities, and recognition programs for individual clinical practices.

Origins and Scope

The NCQA began evaluating and accrediting managed care organizations in 1991 in response to the need for standardized, objective information about the quality of these organizations. Since then, it has expanded the range of organizations that it accredits or certifies to include human subject research protection programs, managed behavioral health care organizations, credentials verification organizations, physician organizations, and others. NCQA has also developed, in collaboration with organizations such as the American Diabetes Association and American Heart Association/American Stroke Association, recognition programs that evaluate and report on the quality of care at the individual physician level.

MCO Accreditation

The NCQA accreditation process is best illustrated by its MCO (managed care organization) accreditation program. More than 75% of individuals enrolled in HMOs are in plans currently accredited by NCQA. Organizations seeking NCQA accreditation must report on a Web-based tool (the Interactive Survey System) their adherence to standards that evaluate the health plan's clinical and administrative systems, including efforts to continuously improve the quality of care and service it delivers. In addition, plans are required to report, and are scored on their performance on, a set (Health Plan Employer Data and Information Set or HEDIS®) of clinical quality measures (see below).

Plans are reviewed against and scored on more than 50 standards and on clinical measures in the following categories:

- Quality improvement
- Credentialing
- Members' rights and responsibilities
- Preventive health services
- Utilization management
- Medical records
- Performance on HEDIS measures

NCQA accreditation surveys are conducted by teams of physicians and managed care experts. A national oversight committee of physicians analyzes the team's findings and assigns one of five possible accreditation levels (excellent, commendable, accredited, provisional, or denied) based on the plan's level of compliance with NCQA standards. NCQA's MCO accreditation process is thus unique among accreditation programs in its use of direct measures of clinical performance in scoring of accreditation.

Recognition Programs

In response to the demand for evaluation of ambulatory care quality, NCQA developed, in partnership with the ADA, a Diabetes Physician Recognition Program® (DPRP) and with the AHA/ASA Heart-Stroke Recognition Program® (HSRP). It has also developed a recognition program (the Physician Practice Connections® program or PPC) that examines the degree to which an office practice has incorporated systems (such as registries, care management, etc) into the practice. Thresholds for achieving recognition in each of the programs are set by expert panels of clinicians and others. Practices that wish to receive recognition submit data and documentation to NCQA, which evaluates the data against the predetermined threshold values. The NCQA recognition programs have been adopted by a number of pay for performance initiatives, including the GE-led Bridges to Excellence® program. A variety of other recognition programs are currently in development.

Performance Measurement

HEDIS® and related NCQA Clinical Measures

NCQA manages the most widely used set of performance measurements for evaluating quality in ambulatory care, HEDIS®. This measurement set, which includes more than 75 fully specified and standardized measures, is used to evaluate health care quality aggregated at the health plans level. NCQA has also created a companion set of measures for use in reporting at the physician office practice level, including those used in the various physician recognition programs. All of the physician-level measures have been submitted to the National Quality Forum (NQF) and have either been endorsed or are in the process of review.

Work related to measurement has led NCQA to develop projects and programs related to distribution and reporting of performance data, ensuring data accuracy, and making sure the performance data are useful to help guide choice.

In summary, NCQA's work in the area of health care evaluation focuses on four key areas: accreditation, recognition programs, data audit oversight, and collection of HEDIS® and related measures. NCQA publicly reports performance data through Quality Compass® (a national database of HEDIS® data and accreditation information) as well as various other evaluation reports for physicians, plans, consumers, and purchasers.

Contact Information

National Committee for Quality Assurance
2000 L St, NW, Ste 500
Washington, DC 20036
202 955-3500
202 955-3599 Fax
www.ncqa.org

Administrators in Medicine

Administrators in Medicine (AIM), a not-for-profit organization, is the national organization for state medical and osteopathic board executives. Founded in 1984, AIM has the mission of assisting and supporting administrators for medical licensing and regulatory authorities to achieve administrative excellence and ultimately advance public safety. AIM offers educational, research, and online services for its members. AIM's public outreach is via the online search engine it provides along with board Web links on its nationally recognized *AIM DocFinder* Web site.

Education is the cornerstone of what AIM does as an organization for member board executives. AIM sponsors a number of educational seminars, including AIM Regional Meetings, where board executives discuss operational issues. Its AIM Institute Educational Workshops—Physician Licensing, Profiles and Technology—provide an excellent overview of best practices and how to avoid pitfalls and are presented by an expert faculty of board senior staff and experts from the credentialing and technology fields. Its Annual Meeting educational program provides an opportunity to hear from national experts in a variety of fields impacting medical licensure and discipline.

AIM's 2007 project, *State Medical Board Investigator Certification Program*, seeks to address the need for highly trained medical board investigators. AIM will create a specialized, focused training program that will provide education and resources for individuals conducting investigations for state medical and osteopathic boards. It will be a well-rounded program that includes basic investigation techniques as well as exposure to the entire system of medical licensure and discipline.

The AIM DocFinder

Celebrating its 10th anniversary in 2006, the AIM *DocFinder* was the only online physician directory of its kind when it was launched in 1996. The *DocFinder* is still recognized for its easy-to-use search engine. *DocFinder* remains the only combined database of all licensing jurisdictions that has its direct source of data from and is controlled by state licensing boards and remains free of charge to the public.

DocFinder contains the licensing background and disciplinary information of physicians and other health care practitioners, in addition to physician profile information from states that have passed physician profile laws. Popular with consumers, *DocFinder* has been featured in numerous state and national publications such as *Newsweek* and *The Wall Street Journal* as well as national and local news broadcasts. Access the AIM *DocFinder* at: www.docboard.org.

Appendixes

Appendix A

Boards of Medical Examiners in the United States and Possessions

Updated June 29, 2006

Larry D Dixon, Executive Administrator
Alabama State Board of Medical Examiners
848 Washington Ave
PO Box 946
Montgomery, AL 36101-0946
334 242-4116
334 242-4155 Fax
E-mail: Ldixon@albme.org
www.albme.org

Leslie G Gallant, Executive Administrator
Alaska State Medical Board
Division of Occupational Licensing
550 W Seventh Ave, Ste 1500
Anchorage, AK 99501
907 269-8163
907 269-8196 Fax
E-mail: Leslie_Gallant@dced.state.ak.us
www.dced.state.ak.us/occ/pmed.htm

Timothy C Miller, Executive Director
Arizona Medical Board
9545 E Doubletree Ranch Rd
Scottsdale, AZ 85258
480 551-2700
480 551-2704 Fax
www.azmdboard.org

Peggy Pryor Cryer, Executive Secretary
Arkansas State Medical Board
2100 Riverfront Dr
Little Rock, AR 72202-1793
501 296-1802
501 603-3555 Fax
E-mail: regdis@armedicalboard.org
www.armedicalboard.org

David T Thornton, Executive Director
Medical Board of California
1426 Howe Ave, Ste 54
Sacramento, CA 95825-3236
916 263-2389
916 263-2387 Fax
www.medbd.ca.gov

Cheryl Hara, PA, JD, Program Administrator
Colorado Board of Medical Examiners
1560 Broadway, Ste 1300
Denver, CO 80202-5140
303 894-7690
303 894-7692 Fax
E-mail: cheryl.hara@dora.state.co.us
www.dora.state.co.us/medical

Jeff Kardys, Board Liaison
Connecticut Medical Examining Board
Physician Licensure Unit
PO Box 340308, 410 Capital Ave, MS #13PHO
Hartford, CT 06134-0308
860 509-7648
860 509-7553 Fax
www.dph.state.ct.us

Gayle MacAfee, Executive Director
Delaware Board of Medical Practice
861 Silver Lake Blvd, Ste 203
Dover, DE 19901
302 739-4520
302 739-2711 Fax
E-mail: gayle.macafee@state.de.us
www.professionallicensing.state.de.us

James R Granger, Jr, Executive Director
District of Columbia Board of Medicine
Health Professional Licensing Administration
717 14th St NW, Ste 600
Washington, DC 20005
202 724-4900
E-mail: jgranger@dchealth.com
www.dchealth.dc.gov

Larry J McPherson, Executive Director
Florida Board of Medicine
Bin # C03
4052 Bald Cypress Way
Tallahassee, FL 32399
850 245-4131
850 488-9325 Fax
www.doh.state.fl.us

LaSharn Hughes, Executive Director
Georgia Composite State Board of Medical Examiners
2 Peachtree Street NW, 36th Fl
Atlanta, GA 30303
404 656-3913
404 656-9723 Fax
E-mail: lhughes@dch.state.ga.us
www.medicalboard.state.ga.us/bdsearch/index.html

Roma C Basa, Acting Administrator
Guam Board of Medical Examiners
PO Box 2816
Hagatna, GU 96932
671 735-7408
671 735-7413 Fax
E-mail: rebasa@dphss.govguam.net

Constance Cabral, Executive Director
Hawaii Board of Medical Examiners
1010 Richards St
PO Box 3469
Honolulu, HI 96813
808 586-3000
808 586-2874 Fax
www.ehawaii.gov

Nancy M Kerr, Executive Director
Idaho State Board of Medicine
1755 Westgate Dr, Ste 140
Boise, ID 83704
208 327-7000
208 327-7005 Fax
www.bom.state.id.us

Sandra Dunn, Board Liaison
Illinois Medical Licensing Board
Department of Professional Regulation
320 W Washington, 3rd Fl
Springfield, IL 62786
217 567-3209
217 524-2169 Fax
E-mail: sdunn@idfpr.com
www.idfpr.com

Michael Rinebold, Executive Director
Indiana Health Professions Bureau
402 W Washington St, Rm 072
Indianapolis, IN 46204
317 232-2960
317 233-4236 Fax
E-mail: MRinebold@pla.in.gov
www.in.gov/hpb

Ann E Mowery, PhD, Executive Director
Iowa Board of Medical Examiners
400 SW 8th St, Ste C
Des Moines, IA 50309-4686
515 281-5171
515 242-5908 Fax
E-mail: ann.mowery@iowa.gov
www.docboard.org/ia/ia_home.htm

Lawrence T Buening, Jr, JD, Executive Director
Kansas Board of Healing Arts
235 S Topeka Blvd
Topeka, KS 66603-3068
785 296-3680
785 296-0852 Fax
E-mail: lbuening@ink.org
www.ksbha.org

C William Schmidt, Executive Director
Kentucky Board of Medical Licensure
Hurstbourne Office Park
310 Whittington Pkwy, Ste 1B
Louisville, KY 40222-4916
502 429-7150
502 429-9923 Fax
E-mail: Bill.Schmidt@ky.gov
www.state.ky.us/agencies/kbml

Robert Marier, MD, Executive Director
Louisiana State Board of Medical Examiners
630 Camp St
PO Box 30250
New Orleans, LA 70190-0250
504 568-6820
504 568-8893 Fax
www.lsbme.louisiana.gov

Randal C Manning, Executive Director
Maine Board of Licensure in Medicine
137 State House Station
Augusta, ME 04333
207 287-3601
207 287-6590 Fax
www.docboard.org/me/me_home.htm

C Irving Pinder, Executive Director
Maryland Board of Physicians
PO Box 2571
4201 Patterson Ave, 3rd Fl
Baltimore, MD 21215-0095
410 764-4777
410 358-2252 Fax
E-mail: mbp@erols.com
www.mbp.state.md.us

Nancy Achin Audesse, Executive Director
Massachusetts Board of Registration in Medicine
560 Harrison Avenue, Ste G-4
Boston, MA 02118
617 654-9800
617 451-9568 Fax
www.massmedboard.org

Rae Ramsdell, Licensing Director
Michigan Board of Medicine
611 W Ottawa St, 1st Fl
PO Box 30670
Lansing, MI 48933
517 373-6873
517 373-2179 Fax
E-mail: rhramsd@michigan.gov
www.michigan.gov/cis

Robert A Leach, JD, Executive Director
Minnesota Board of Medical Practice
University Park Plaza
2829 University Ave SE, Ste 500
Minneapolis, MN 55414-3246
612 617-2130
612 617-2166 Fax
www.bmp.state.mn.us

Mallan G Morgan, MD, Executive Director
Mississippi State Board of Medical Licensure
1867 Crane Ridge Dr, Ste 200B
Jackson, MS 39216
601 987-3079
601 987-4159 Fax
E-mail: mboard@msbml.state.ms.us
www.msbml.state.ms.us

Tina M Steinman, Executive Director
Missouri State Board of Registration for the Healing Arts
Division of Professional Registration
3605 Missouri Blvd
Jefferson City, MO 65109
573 751-0098
573 751-3166 Fax
E-mail: tina.steinman@pr.mo.gov
www.pr.mo.gov/healingarts.asp

Jeannie I Worsech, Executive Director
Montana Board of Medical Examiners
PO Box 200513
301 S Park Ave, 4th Fl
Helena, MT 59620-0513
406 841-2364
406 841-2305 Fax
www.medical board.mt.gov

Becky A Wisell, Section Administrator
Nebraska Board of Medicine and Surgery
Regulation and Licensure Credentialing Division
301 Centennial Mall South, PO Box 94986
Lincoln, NE 68509-4986
402 471-2118
402 471-3577 Fax
E-mail: becky.wisell@hhs.state.ne.us
www.hhs.state.ne.us

Drennan A Clark, JD, Executive Secretary/Special Counsel
Nevada State Board of Medical Examiners
Ste 301, 1105 Terminal Way
Reno, NV 89502
775 688-2559
775 688-2321 Fax
E-mail: nsbme@medboard.nv.gov
www.medboard.nv.gov

Penny Taylor, Administrator
New Hampshire Board of Medicine
2 Industrial Park Dr, Ste 8
Concord, NH 03301-8520
603 271-1205
603 271-6702 Fax
E-mail: ptaylor@nhsa.state.nh.us
www.state.nh.us/medicine

William J Roeder, Executive Director
New Jersey State Board of Medical Examiners
PO Box 183
140 E Front Street, 2nd Fl
Trenton, NJ 08608
609 826-7100
609 826-7117 Fax
www.state.nj.us/lps/ca/medical.htm#bme5

Lynn S Hart, Executive Director
New Mexico Medical Board
2055 S Pacheco St, Building 400
Santa Fe, NM 87505
505 476-7220
505 476-7233 Fax
E-mail: lynns.hart@state.nm.us
www.state.nm.us/nmbme

Thomas J Monahan, Executive Secretary
New York State Board for Medicine
89 Washington Ave
2nd Fl West Wing
Albany, NY 12234
518 474-3817
518 486-4846 Fax
E-mail: tmonahan@mail.nysed.gov
www.op.nysed.gov

R David Henderson, JD, Executive Director
North Carolina Medical Board
1203 Front St
PO Box 20007
Raleigh, NC 27619
919 326-1100
919 326-1131 Fax
E-mail: david.henderson@ncmedboard.org
www.ncmedboard.org

Rolf P Sletten, JD, Executive Secretary and Treasurer
North Dakota State Board of Medical Examiners
418 E Broadway Ave, Ste 12
Bismarck, ND 58501
701 328-6500
701 328-6505 Fax
E-mail: bomex@tic.bisman.com
www.ndbomex.com

Richard A Whitehouse, JD, Executive Director
State Medical Board of Ohio
77 S High St, 17th Fl
Columbus, OH 43215
614 466-3934
614 728-5946 Fax
E-mail: Richard.Whitehouse@med.state.oh.us
www.med.ohio.gov

Lyle Kelsey, CAE, Executive Director
Oklahoma State Board of Medical Licensure and Supervision
PO Box 18256
Oklahoma City, OK 73118
405 848-6841
405 848-4999 Fax
E-mail: lkelsey@okmedicalboard.org
www.okmedicalboard.org

Kathleen Haley, JD, Executive Director
Oregon Board of Medical Examiners
1500 SW First Ave
620 Crown Plaza
Portland, OR 97201-5826
971 673-2713
971 673-2672 Fax
E-mail: kathleen.haley@state.or.us
www.oregon.gov/bme

Tammy Radel, Administrator
Pennsylvania State Board of Medicine
2601N Third St, PO Box 2649
Harrisburg, PA 17105-2649
717 787-7768
717 787-7769 Fax
E-mail: st-medicine@state.pa.us
www.dos.state.pa.us

Pablo M Valentin-Torres, Executive Director
Board of Medical Examiners of Puerto Rico
PO Box 13969
San Juan, PR 00908
787 782-8937
787 792-4436 Fax

Robert S Crausman, MD, Chief Administrator
Rhode Island Board of Medical Licensure and Discipline
Cannon Bldg, Rm 205
Three Capitol Hill
Providence, RI 02908-5097
401 222-3855
401 222-2158 Fax
E-mail: RobertC@doh.state.ri.us
www.health.ri.gov/hsr/bmld

Bruce Duke, Board Administrator
South Carolina Board of Medical Examiners
Department of Labor, Licensing & Regulation
110 Centerview Dr, Ste 202
Columbia, SC 29210-1289
803 896-4500
803 896-4515 Fax
E-mail: medboard@llr.sc.gov
www.llr.state.sc.us/pol/medical

Margaret B Hansen, Executive Director
South Dakota State Board of Medical & Osteopathic Examiners
123 S Main Ave, Ste 100
Sioux Falls, SD 57104
605 367-7781
605 367-7786 Fax
E-mail: margaret.hansen@state.sd.us
www.state.sd.us/dcr/medical

Rosemarie Otto, Executive Director
Tennessee Board of Medical Examiners
First Fl, Cordell Hull Bldg
425 5th Ave North
Nashville, TN 37247-1010
615 532-3202
615 253-4484 Fax
E-mail: rosemarie.otto@state.tn.us
www.state.tn.us/health

Donald W Patrick, MD, JD, Executive Director
Texas Medical Board
PO Box 2018
Austin, TX 78768-2018
512 305-7010
512 305-7051 Fax
www.tmb.state.tx.us

Craig Jackson, RPh, Director
State of Utah Department of Commerce
Division of Occupational & Professional Licensure
Heber M Wells Building, 4th Fl, 160 East 300 South
Salt Lake City, UT 84114-6741
801 530-6628
801 530-6511 Fax
E-mail: cjackson@utah.gov
www.dopl.utah.gov

Paula J DiStabile, Executive Director
Vermont Board of Medical Practice
108 Cherry St, PO Box 70
Burlington, VT 05402-0070
802 657-4220
802 657-4227 Fax
http://healthvermont.gov/hc/med_board/bmp.aspx

William Harp, MD, Executive Director
Virginia Board of Medicine
6603 W Broad St, 5th Fl
Richmond, VA 23230
804 662-9908
804 662-9517 Fax
E-mail: medbd@dhp.state.va.us
www.dhp.state.va.us/medicine

Lydia Scott, Executive Assistant
Virgin Islands Board of Medical Examiners
Office of the Commissioner, Department of Health
48 Sugar Estate
St Thomas, VI 00802
340 774-0117
340 777-4001 Fax
E-mail: Lydia.Scott@usvi-doh.org

Blake T Maresh, MPA, Executive Director
Washington Medical Quality Assurance Commission
Department of Health
PO Box 47866
Olympia, WA 98504-7866
360 236-4790
360 236-4768 Fax
E-mail: blake.maresh@doh.wa.gov
www.doh.wa.gov

Robert D Knittle, Executive Director
West Virginia Board of Medicine
101 Dee Dr
Charleston, WV 25311
304 558-2921
304 558-2084 Fax
E-mail: bobknittle@wvdhhr.org
www.wvdhhr.org/wvbom

Thomas D Ryan, Bureau Director
State of Wisconsin Medical Examining Board
Dept of Regulation & Licensing
1400 E Washington Ave
Madison, WI 53703
608 266-8098
608 261-7083 Fax
E-mail: thomas.ryan@drl.state.wi.us
http://drl.wi.gov/index.htm

Carole Shotwell, JD, Executive Secretary
Wyoming Board of Medicine
Colony Bldg, 2nd Fl
211 W 19th St
Cheyenne, WY 82002
307 778-7053
307 778-2069 Fax
E-mail: wyobom@aol.com
http://wyomedboard.state.wy.us

Appendix B

Boards of Osteopathic Medical Examiners in the United States and Possessions

Updated June 29, 2006

Jack Confer, Executive Director
Arizona Board of Osteopathic Examiners in Medicine & Surgery
9535 E Doubletree Ranch Rd
Scottsdale, AZ 85258-5539
480 657-7703
480 657-7715 Fax
E-mail: Executive.Director@azosteoboard.org
www.azosteoboard.org

Angelina Burton, Acting Executive Director
Osteopathic Medical Board of California
2720 Gateway Oaks Dr, Ste 350
Sacramento, CA 95833-3500
916 263-3100
916 263-3117 Fax
E-mail: angie_burton@dca.ca.gov
www.dca.ca.gov/osteopathic

Pamela D King, Executive Director
Florida Board of Osteopathic Medicine
Bin #C06
4052 Bald Cypress Way
Tallahassee, FL 32399-1753
850 245-4161
850 487-9874 Fax
www.doh.state.fl.us/mqa

Susan E Strout, Executive Secretary
Maine Board of Osteopathic Licensure
142 State House Station
Augusta, ME 04333-0142
207 287-2480
207 287-3015 Fax
E-mail: susan.e.strout@maine.gov
www.maine.gov/osteo

Rae Ramsdell, Licensing Director
Michigan Board of Osteopathic Medicine & Surgery
611 W Ottawa St, 1st Fl
Lansing, MI 48933
517 373-6873
517 373-2179 Fax
E-mail: rhramsd@michigan.gov
www.michigan.gov/cis

Larry J Tarno, DO, Executive Director
Nevada State Board of Osteopathic Medicine
2860 E Flamingo Rd, Ste D
Las Vegas, NV 89121
702 732-2147
702 732-2079 Fax
www.osteo.state.nv.us

Liz King, Board Administrator
New Mexico Board of Osteopathic Medical Examiners
2550 Cerrillos Rd
Santa Fe, NM 87505
505 476-4695
505 476-4545 Fax
E-mail: osteopathic.board@state.nm.us
www.rld.state.nm.us/b&c/osteopathic_examiners_board.htm

Gary R Clark, Executive Director
Oklahoma Board of Osteopathic Examiners
4848 N Lincoln Blvd, Ste 100
Oklahoma City, OK 73105-3321
405 528-8625
405 557-0653 Fax
E-mail: okosteoexaminers@aol.com
www.docboard.org

Gina Bittner, Administrator
Pennsylvania State Board of Osteopathic Medicine
124 Pine St
PO Box 2649
Harrisburg, PA 17101
717 783-4858
717 787-7769 Fax
E-mail: gbittner@state.pa.us
www.dos.state.pa.us

Rosemarie Otto, Executive Director
Tennessee State Board of Osteopathic Examiners
First Fl, Cordell Hull Bldg
425 5th Avenue North
Nashville, TN 37247-1010
615 741-4540
615 253-4484 Fax
E-mail: rosemarie.otto@state.tn.us
www.state.tn.us/health

Diana Baker, Bureau Manager
State of Utah Department of Commerce
Division of Occupational & Professional Licensing, Osteopathic
PO Box 146741, 160 East 300 South
Salt Lake City, UT 84114-6741
801 530-6179
801 530-6511 Fax
E-mail: dbaker@utah.gov
www.dopl.utah.gov

Christopher D Winters, Director
Vermont Board of Osteopathic Physicians and Surgeons
Vermont Section of State Office, Office of Professional Regulations
26 Terrace Street, Drawer 09
Montpelier, VT 05609-1106
802 828-2373
802 828-2465 Fax
http://vtprofessionals.org/opr1/osteopaths

Blake Maresh, Executive Director
Washington Board of Osteopathic Medicine & Surgery
Department of Health
PO Box 47866
Olympia, WA 98504-7866
360 236-4945
360 236-2406 Fax
https://fortress.wa.gov/doh/hpqa1/HPS7/Osteopath/default.htm

Cheryl E Schreiber, Executive Secretary
West Virginia Board of Osteopathy
334 Penco Rd
Weirton, WV 26062
304 723-4638
304 723-2877 Fax
www.wvbdosteo.org

Appendix C

Member Organizations of the Federation of Medical Regulatory Authorities of Canada

Updated June 20, 2006

Fleur-Ange Lefebvre, Executive Director and CEO
Federation of Medical Regulatory Authorities of Canada
2283 St Laurent Blvd
Ottawa, ON K1G 5A2
613 738-0372
613 738-9169 Fax
www.fmrac.ca

Trevor Theman, MD, Registrar
College of Physicians and Surgeons of Alberta
900 Manulife Pl, 10180-101 St
Edmonton, AB T5J 4P8
780 423-4764
780 420-0651 Fax
www.cpsa.ab.ca

Morris Vanandel, MD, Registrar
College of Physicians and Surgeons of British Columbia
400-858 Beatty St
Vancouver, BC V6B 1C1
604 733-3503
604 733-1047 Fax
www.cpsbc.ca

William Pope, MD, Registrar
College of Physicians and Surgeons of Manitoba
1000-1661 Portage Ave
Winnipeg, MB R3J 3T7
204 774-4344
204 774-0750 Fax
www.cpsm.mb.ca

Edmund Schollenberg, MD, Registrar
College of Physicians and Surgeons of New Brunswick
One Hampton Rd, Ste 300
Rothesay, NB E2E 5K8
506 849-5050
506 849-5069 Fax
www.cpsnb.org

Robert W. Young, MD, Registrar
College of Physicians and Surgeons of Newfoundland and Labrador
139 Water St, St John's, NF A1C 1B2
709 726-8546
709 726-4725 Fax
E-mail: ryoung@cpsnl.ca
www.cpsnl.ca

Cameron Little, MD, Registrar
College of Physicians and Surgeons of Nova Scotia
200-1559 Brunswick St, Sentry Place
Halifax, NS B3J 2G1
902 422-5823
902 422-5035 Fax
www.cpsns.ns.ca

Ben Van Den Assem, Registrar, Professional Services
Department of Health and Social Services
Government of Nunavut
Box 390
Kugluktuk, NU X0B 0E0
867 982-7668
867 982-3256 Fax
E-mail: bvandenassem@gov.nu.ca

Jeannette Hall, Registrar
Department of Health and Social Service
Government of the Northwest Territories
Centre Square Tower
5022 49th St, 8th Fl, PO Box 1320
Yellowknife, NWT X1A 2L9
867 920-8058
867 873-0281 Fax
E-mail: jeannette_hall@gov.nt.ca

Rocco Gerace, MD, Registrar
College of Physicians and Surgeons of Ontario
80 College St
Toronto, ON M5G 2E2
416 967-2600 or 800 268-7096
416 961-3330 Fax
www.cpso.on.ca

Cyril Moyse, MD, Registrar
College of Physicians and Surgeons of Prince Edward Island
199 Grafton St
Charlottetown, PEI C1A 1L2
902 566-3861
902 566-3861 Fax
E-mail: mmacdonald@collegeofphysicians.pe.ca

Yves Robert, MD, Secrétaire-général
College des médecins du Québec
2170 boul René Lévésque ouest
Montréal, PQ H3H 2T8
514 933-4441
514 933-3112 Fax
www.cmq.org

Dennis A. Kendel, MD, Registrar
College of Physicians and Surgeons of Saskatchewan
211 4th Ave S
Saskatoon, SK S7K 1N1
306 244-7355
306 244-0090 Fax
www.quadrant.net/cpss

Dale Kozmen, Registrar
Department of Community Services
Government of the Yukon
2130 Second Ave, 3rd Fl
PO Box 2703
Whitehorse, YT Y1A 2C6
867 667-5828
867 393-6249 Fax
E-mail: dale.kozmen@gov.yk.ca

Appendix D

Glossary of Medical Licensure Terms

Accreditation Council for Graduate Medical Education (ACGME)

Note: See p. 123 for more information.

An accrediting agency with the mission of improving the quality of health in the United States by ensuring and improving the quality of allopathic graduate medical education for physicians in training. The ACGME establishes national standards for graduate medical education by which it approves and continually assesses educational programs under its aegis. The ACGME accredits GME programs through its 28 review committees (26 Residency Review Committees, or RRCs, the Transitional Year Review Committee, and the Institutional Review Committee). The ACGME has five member organizations:

- American Board of Medical Specialties
- American Hospital Association
- American Medical Association
- Association of American Medical Colleges
- Council of Medical Specialty Societies

Each member organization nominates four directors. In addition, the ACGME Board of Directors includes two resident physician member, the Chair of the Council of Review Committee Chairs, and three public members. A federal government representative also serves on the board in a non-voting capacity.

American Board of Medical Specialties (ABMS®)

Note: See p. 120 for more information.

A nonprofit organization of 24 approved medical specialty boards. Its mission is to maintain and improve the quality of medical care by helping its member boards develop and use professional and educational standards for the evaluation and certification of physician specialists. The certification of physicians provides assurance to the public that a physician specialist certified by an ABMS member board has successfully completed an approved educational program and an evaluation process that assesses the knowledge, skills, and experience required to provide quality patient care in that specialty. Medical specialty board certification is an additional process to receiving a medical degree, completing residency training, and receiving a license to practice medicine.

Boards and certification

Note: See p. 123 for more information.

Each medical specialty (as defined by the ABMS) has its own unique Board examination process. This process is voluntary and is intended to assure the public that a certified medical specialist has successfully completed an approved educational program and an evaluation including an examination process designed to assess the knowledge, experience, and skills requisite to the provision of high-quality patient care in that specialty.

General board certification is the first certification awarded by an ABMS member board to approved candidates who meet the requirements for certification in a specified field of medical practice.

Subspecialty board certification is conferred by one or more ABMS member boards in a component of a specialty or subspecialty. It is conferred only to certified medical specialists who have been certified by one or more member boards in an area of general certification.

Some ABMS member boards also issue *certificates of added qualifications* or *certificates of special qualifications.* (Source: ABMS)

Also see "Maintenance of Certification."

Clerkship

Note: See p. 32 for more information.

Clinical education provided to medical students. Table 10 contains information on clerkship regulations of state medical boards.

Clinical Skills Assessment (CSA)

A 1-day exam, formerly administered by the ECFMG, that required examinees to demonstrate both clinical proficiency and spoken English language proficiency. Step 2 Clinical Skills (Step 2 CS) of the USMLE is the exam currently administered that satisfies the clinical skills requirement for ECFMG Certification.

Also see "Step 2 CS."

Comprehensive Osteopathic Medical Licensing Examination (COMLEX)

Note: See p. 94 for more information.

A three-level examination initiated in 1995 by the National Board of Osteopathic Medical Examiners to replace the former three-part NBOME examination series and to better assist the state licensing boards in measuring the knowledge required by today's physicians.

The COMLEX program is designed to assess the osteopathic medical knowledge considered essential for osteopathic generalist physicians to practice medicine without supervision. COMLEX is constructed in the context of medical problem solving, which involves clinical presentations and physician tasks.

ECFMG number

Note: See p. 98 for more information.

The number assigned by the Educational Commission for Foreign Medical Graduates (ECFMG) to each international medical graduate (IMG) who applies for certification from ECFMG. Almost all graduates of foreign medical schools must have an ECFMG certificate to participate in graduate medical education in the United States.

Educational Commission for Foreign Medical Graduates (ECFMG)

Note: See p. 98 for more information.

A nonprofit organization that assesses the readiness of graduates of foreign medical schools to enter residency programs in the United States accredited by the Accreditation Council for Graduate Medical Education (ACGME).

ECFMG certification provides assurance to directors of ACGME-accredited residency programs, and to the people of the United States, that graduates of foreign medical schools have met minimum standards of eligibility required to enter such programs. This certification does not guarantee that such graduates will be accepted into these programs in the United States, since the number of applicants frequently exceeds the number of positions available.

ECFMG certification is also a prerequisite required by most states for licensure to practice medicine in the United States and is one of the eligibility requirements to take Step 3 of the United States Medical Licensing Examination (USMLE).

Endorsement, licensure

Note: See p. 11 for more information.

A process through which a state issues an unrestricted license to practice medicine to an individual who holds a valid and unrestricted license in another jurisdiction. Licensure endorsement is generally based on documentation of successfully completing approved examinations, authentication of required core documents, and completion of any additional requirements assessing the applicant's fitness to practice medicine in the new jurisdiction. Previously referred to as "reciprocity."

Fellow

A. A physician in an ACGME-accredited program that is beyond the requirements for eligibility for first board certification in the discipline. Such physicians may also be termed "resident" as well. Other uses of the term "fellow" require modifiers for precision and clarity, eg, "research fellow."
   Also see "Resident or resident physician."

B. A physician who has demonstrated outstanding achievements in medicine, usually within a given medical specialty society. Typical criteria for fellowship in a specialty society include years of membership, years as a practitioner in the specialty, and professional recognition by peers.

Federation Licensing Examination (FLEX)

Note: See p. 11 for more information.

Originally introduced in 1968 and subsequently enhanced and modified in 1985, this examination was administered for the last time in December 1993. In 1994, the United States Medical Licensing Examination (USMLE) was fully implemented. Some candidates for licensure may have a combination of scores from FLEX and USMLE. *Also see "United States Medical Licensing Examination."*

Federation of State Medical Boards (FSMB)

Note: See p. 88 for more information.

A nonprofit organization whose membership comprises the allopathic, osteopathic, and composite medical licensing boards of all the states, the District of Columbia, Guam, Puerto Rico, and the Virgin Islands. Its primary responsibility is to protect the public through the regulation of physicians and other health care providers. It serves as a liaison, advocate, and information source to the public, health care organizations, and state, national, and international authorities. The FSMB promotes high standards for physician licensure and practice and assists and supports state medical boards collectively and individually in the regulation of medical practice and in their role of public protection.

Fifth Pathway

Note: See p. 28 for more information.

One of several ways that individuals who obtain their undergraduate medical education abroad can enter GME in the United States. The Fifth Pathway is a period of supervised clinical training for students who obtained their premedical education in the United States, received undergraduate medical education abroad, and passed Step 1 of the United States Medical Licensing Examination. After these students successfully complete a year of clinical training sponsored by a US medical school accredited by the Liaison Committee on Medical Education (LCME) and pass USMLE Step 2, they receive a Fifth Pathway certificate and become eligible for an ACGME-accredited residency as an international medical graduate. Currently, New York Medical College in Valhalla, NY, is the primary medical school that offers the Fifth Pathway.

FLEX Weighted Average (FWA)

Note: See p. 11 for more information.

All states currently require a minimum passing score of 75 on each component of the post-1985 two-part FLEX; the resulting number composes the Federation Licensing Examination (FLEX) Weighted Average.

Initial license

Note: See p. 74 for more information.

The first ever full and unrestricted license a physician receives in his/her medical career. Some medical boards interpret "initial license" as a physician's first license in their particular states (although the physician could already have been licensed in other states). This publication does not use the term in this sense.

Intern

No longer used by the AMA or ACGME. Historically, "intern" was used to designate individuals in the first post-MD year of hospital training; less commonly, it designated individuals in the first year of any residency program. Since 1975, the AMA's *Graduate Medical Education Directory* and the ACGME have used "resident," "resident physician," or "fellow" to designate all individuals in ACGME-accredited programs. *Also see "Resident or resident physician" and "Fellow."*

International medical graduate (IMG)

A graduate from a medical school outside of the United States and Canada. Formerly referred to as "foreign medical graduate" (FMG).

Liaison Committee on Medical Education (LCME)

The body that accredits educational programs in the United States and Canada leading to the MD degree. The American Osteopathic Association (AOA) accredits educational programs leading to the doctor of osteopathy (DO) degree.

Licensure

The process by which a state or jurisdiction of the United States admits physicians to the practice of medicine. Licensure ensures that practicing physicians have appropriate education and training and that they abide by recognized standards of professional conduct while serving their patients. Candidates for first licensure must complete a rigorous examination designed to assess a physician's ability to apply knowledge, concepts, and principles that are important in health and disease and that constitute the basis of safe and effective patient care. All applicants must submit proof of medical education and training and provide details about their work history. Finally, applicants may have to reveal information regarding past medical history (including the use of habit-forming drugs and emotional or mental illness), arrests, and convictions. *Also see "Limited license" and "Reregistration."*

Limited license

Note: See p. 56 for more information.

Issued by state medical boards to resident physicians in graduate medical education (GME) programs within their jurisdictions. Physicians do not receive a full and unrestricted license until completion of GME and fulfillment of other licensure requirements in a given jurisdiction.

Locum tenens

This Latin term (locum "place," tenens "to hold") describes a person taking another's place for the time being. In medicine, for example, the American Medical Association's Project USA provides short-term replacements for US Public Health Service physicians in rural locations, allowing them to take a vacation or fulfill continuing medical education requirements (see "Project USA," p. 131).

Maintenance of Certification

Note: See p. 120 for more information.

To better evaluate the competence of physician specialists throughout their careers, ABMS Member Boards are moving from "recertification" to a more comprehensive plan called "maintenance of certification." Where recertification programs evaluate physicians every 7 to 10 years, primarily by a written examination, Maintenance of Certification© is an in-depth program that will be continuous and relevant to practice. A key component of this program is the evaluation of physician practice performance, including six core competencies (patient care, medical knowledge, interpersonal and communication skills, professionalism, practice-based learning and improvement, and systems-based practice).

Medical Practice Act

A statute of a US state or jurisdiction that outlines the practice of medicine and the responsibility of the medical board to regulate that practice. The primary responsibility and obligation of a state medical board is to protect the public through proper licensing and regulation of physicians and, in some jurisdictions, other health care professionals. *Also see "Unprofessional conduct."*

National Board of Medical Examiners (NBME)

Note: See p. 92 for more information.

A nonprofit, independent organization that prepares and administers medical qualifying examinations, either independently or jointly with other organizations. Legal agencies governing the practice of medicine within each US state or jurisdiction may grant a license without further examination for those physicians who have successfully completed such examinations and met other requirements.

Currently, the NBME administers USMLE Steps 1 and 2 to students and graduates of US and Canadian medical and osteopathic schools accredited by the Liaison Committee on Medical Education or the American Osteopathic Association.

National Board of Osteopathic Medical Examiners (NBOME)

Note: See p. 94 for more information.

A not-for-profit corporation serving the public and state licensing agencies by administering examinations testing the medical knowledge of those who seek to practice as osteopathic physicians.

The NBOME examinations have been the primary pathway by which osteopathic physicians have applied for licensure to practice osteopathic medicine. A passing score on these examinations verifies a student's adequacy of medical knowledge for practicing osteopathic medicine.

Reregistration

Note: See p. 63 for more information.

After physicians are licensed in a state or jurisdiction, they must reregister periodically to continue their active status. During this reregistration process, physicians are required to demonstrate that they have maintained acceptable standards of ethics and medical practice and have not engaged in improper conduct. In many states, physicians must also show that they have completed a set number of hours of continuing medical education.

Resident or resident physician

Any individual at any level in an ACGME-accredited GME program, including subspecialty programs. Local usage might refer to these individuals as interns, house officers, house staff, trainees, fellows, or other comparable terminology. Beginning in 2000, the ACGME has used the term "fellow" to denote physicians in subspecialty programs (vs residents in specialty programs) or in GME programs that are beyond the requirements for eligibility for first board certification in the discipline.

Also see "Fellow."

Special Purpose Examination (SPEX)

Note: See p. 90 for more information.

This 1-day, computer-administered examination, with approximately 420 multiple-choice questions, assesses primary care medical knowledge and skills. It does not include questions specific to a particular specialty or subspecialty. The SPEX is used to assess physicians who have held a valid, unrestricted license in a US or Canadian jurisdiction who are:

- Required by the state medical board to demonstrate current medical knowledge
- Seeking endorsement licensure some years beyond initial examination
- Seeking license reinstatement after a period of professional inactivity

Physicians holding a valid, unrestricted license may also apply for SPEX, independent of any request or approval from a medical licensing board.

Specialty

A medical specialty is a defined area of medical practice that connotes special knowledge and ability resulting from specialized effort and training in the special field. (Source: ABMS)

Also see "Subspecialty."

Step 2 CS

The Clinical Skills component of USMLE Step 2, in tandem with the Clinical Knowledge component (Step 2 CK), became a part of Step 2 in June 2004. Step 2 assesses whether medical school students and graduates can understand and apply the knowledge, skills, and understanding of clinical science considered essential for the provision of patient care under supervision and includes emphasis on health promotion and disease prevention. The inclusion of Step 2 in the USMLE sequence is intended to ensure that due attention is devoted to principles of clinical sciences and basic patient-centered skills that provide the foundation for safe and competent medical practice.

Subspecialty

A medical subspecialty is an identifiable component of a specialty to which a practicing physician may devote a significant proportion of time. Practice in the subspecialty follows special educational experience in addition to that required for general certification. (*Note:* Two different specialty fields may include two or more similar subspecialty areas, eg, sports medicine as a subspecialty of emergency medicine and family practice. In these cases the identified subspecialty area might use the same title and equivalent educational standards.) (Source: ABMS)

Also see "Specialty."

Telemedicine

Note: See p. 69 for more information.

Telemedicine is the delivery of health care services via electronic means from a health care provider in one location to a patient in another. Applications that fall under this definition include the transfer of medical images, such as pathology slides or radiographs, interactive video consultations between patient and provider or between primary care and specialty care physicians, and mental health consultations.

Unprofessional conduct

Although laws vary from one jurisdiction to the next, the Medical Practice Acts in force in most US jurisdictions would define unprofessional conduct as including:

- Physical abuse of a patient
- Inadequate recordkeeping
- Not recognizing or acting on common symptoms
- Prescribing drugs in excessive amounts or without legitimate reason
- Impaired ability to practice due to addiction or physical or mental illness
- Failing to meet continuing medical education requirements
- Performing duties beyond the scope of a license
- Dishonesty
- Conviction of a felony
- Delegating the practice of medicine to an unlicensed individual

Unprofessional conduct would not include minor disagreements or poor customer service.

United States Medical Licensing Examination (USMLE)

Note: See p. 80 for more information.

This three-step examination for US medical licensure provides a common evaluation system for applicants. The USMLE program is governed by a composite committee of representatives from the Federation of State Medical Boards (FSMB), the National Board of Medical Examiners (NBME), the Educational Commission for Foreign Medical Graduates (ECFMG), and the public.

Results of the USMLE are reported to state medical boards for use in granting the initial license to practice medicine. Each medical licensing authority requires, as part of its licensing processes, successful completion of an examination or other certification demonstrating qualification for licensure.

The USMLE replaced FLEX and the certifying examination of the NBME, as well as the Foreign Medical Graduate Examination in the Medical Sciences (FMGEMS), which was formerly used by the ECFMG for certification purposes. Steps 1 and 2 of the USMLE are used as the examination for ECFMG certification. These two steps are also used for promotion and graduation in some US medical schools.